LIVING FROM
THE CENTER WITHIN

Co-Creating Who You Are Becoming

LIVING FROM
THE CENTER WITHIN

Co-Creating Who You Are Becoming

Michele Rae

Paragon House

First Edition 2017

Published in the United States by
Paragon House

www.ParagonHouse.com

Grateful acknowledgment is given for permission to reprint the following copyrighted material:

Hafiz, "Now is the Time," from the Penguin publication *The Gift: Poems by Hafiz* by Daniel Ladinsky. Copyright © 1999 Daniel Ladinsky and used with his permission. #47 from *The Way of Life According to Lao-Tzu* edited by Witter Bynner. Copyright 1944 by Witte Bynner, renewed © 1972 by Dorothy Chavenet and Paul Hogan. Reprinted by permission of HarperCollins Publishers. Mewlana Jalaluddin Rumi, "Out Beyond Ideas," from HarperCollins publication *The Essential Rumi* translated by Coleman Barks Copyright © 2004 HarperCollins and used with his permission. Portia Nelson, "An Autobiography in 5 Short Chapters" from Beyond Words Publishing publication *There's a Hole in My Sidewalk: The Romance of Self-Discovery.* Copyright © 1993 Portia Nelson and used with her permission.

Library of Congress Cataloging-in-Publication Data

Names: Rae, Michele, 1961- author.
Title: Living from the center within : co-creating who we are becoming / by
 Michele Rae.
Description: first [edition]. | Saint Paul, Minnesota : Paragon House, 2017.
 | Includes bibliographical references and index.
Identifiers: LCCN 2016035360 | ISBN 9781557789297 (pbk. : alk. paper)
Subjects: LCSH: Self-actualization (Psychology)
Classification: LCC BF637.S4 .R23 2017 | DDC 158--dc23 LC record available at
https://lccn.loc.gov/2016035360

Manufactured in the United States of America

10 9 8 7 6 5 4 3 2 1

The paper used in this publication meets the minimum requirements of American National Standard for Information Sciences—Permanence of Paper for Printed Library Materials, ANSIZ39.48-1984.

This book is dedicated to my grandchildren Elliana and Odin,
and all the children who will inherit the earth.

ACKNOWLEDGMENTS

With heartfelt gratitude I thank my spiritual directors and teachers along the way. A big "Thank You" to my clients and students who teach me. And to my inner circle of confidants and friends, some who are new in my life and some I have known nearly my entire life, your witness and support in my unfolding process has been priceless. To my children who continuously inspire me, my open heart salutes you.

I am grateful for the expertise and encouragement of my editor Ellie Roscher, and those who have read my manuscripts and provided invaluable feedback, Yvonne, Kendra, and Kim. Thank you Alicia Weller Thompson for the illustrations, Holly Day for the indexing, Lora Matz for the cover photography, Sandra Julian for portrait photography, and Gordon Anderson from Paragon House for your wealth of knowledge. I am deeply appreciative for the financial support from all who donated to my Kickstarter campaign.

CONTENTS

INTRODUCTION

Since I was a small child, I have been fascinated by the interconnection between the seen and unseen world. How did those saints float when they were praying? Why does my body feel so different when I walk in a crowded shopping center versus a walk in my favorite park? Where do insights and revelations come from? My curiosity led me to explore sacred teachings, human development, spiritual practices and many areas of science.

The process of being human is amazing and complex. Why do people having similar experiences react so differently? Some people are resilient, happy, and satisfied, living from their strengths, passions, and gifts. Others with comparable circumstance are miserable and think they are victims. The unseen world of beliefs, intentions, and thoughts have profound influence on the small decisions we make every day.

By paying attention and being mindful, I realized I could move my attention from drama and live with inner peace and contentment. From my calm **Center Within,** I have the freedom to respond to inner and outer knowings and events and make optimal choices in my life. This capacity has shifted my perspective and expanded my worldview and impacts every area of my life. I am more present in the moment and more effective in my roles as parent, leader, lover, coach, teacher, and friend.

This process of discovery of what it means to be a fully realized and awake human is continuous. I have learned to meditate, breathe deeply, and relax. I have walked labyrinths all over the world, learned Reiki and Therapeutic Touch, Qi Gong, and biofeedback. I have studied and practiced emotional and social intelligence, spiritual direction, coaching, intuition, authentic communication, and mind-body skills. I am a lifelong student of being human.

I have been blessed with amazing spiritual teachers, friends, and communities that have and still do share and support my journey. My quest for learning has led me to teach at the Center for Spirituality & Healing at the University of Minnesota where my students challenge and humble me. As a transformational coach and consultant, my individual and organizational clients open me to more clarity and knowledge through sharing their stories of courage, suffering, brilliance, and transformation.

This book, *Living From the Center Within*, arose from invitations by clients and students to make available in written form what we discuss in our sessions and classrooms. It is also in response to the urgency many of us are experiencing as we navigate the accelerating and often confusing changes in our lives and the world. This time of transformation provides an opening and calling to each of us to create a life and a world with more peace, tolerance, and equanimity.

Living From the Center Within is designed to be highly practical, helping you explore and experience the ideas presented. All that is offered is intended to be a working model and a map. This book describes the territory of levels of consciousness and invites you to examine and contemplate your lived experience on your journey through these levels. Some of the ideas may challenge you to go beyond your current belief system and be open to a significantly expanded worldview. Please consider and explore the ideas with an open mind and heart.

Living From the Center Within is also a call to action for personal and societal growth and development. Fortunately, it is our natural tendency to develop. We can actively cultivate our progression. The book has been written as a guide, inviting you to participate with intention, co-creating the emerging paradigms and stories about who we are becoming. It is an invitation for you to contribute to building a world that is abundant and sustainable for all life. It is organized as a self-study guide. Each chapter is followed by questions designed for self-discovery, conversation, and building the reader's capacities for higher consciousness. The ideas in this book can be explored individually or in groups.

The first section of *Living From the Center Within*, "The Way," names concepts and establishes a working vocabulary. The first two chapters articulate that we are shifting to a new era ripe for connectivity and creativity. Change can be scary, but it is also necessary. It is a strategic opportunity to move together toward a higher level of consciousness by living out of a sense of calm and cultivating a peaceful life that actualizes our selves and changes us at the core of our being.

Chapters Three and Four differentiate and explore three main levels of consciousness, each with their own governing properties: **I am Individual, I am Interconnected**, and **I am Infinite**. The first level is living in a sense of isolation, fear, and scarcity. Energy seeps from us. Living in the second level, we live with a sense of wholeness, connectedness, and compassion. The third level is one of pure bliss where we know unity of self and totality.

Chapter Five discusses why expanded consciousness matters. With intentional practice, we can spend more time in higher levels of consciousness to the benefit of all. Service is more effective, art is born, healing and transformation is possible. Seeing ourselves as connected to a web of existence brings with it a life-giving sense of peace. The universe responds, shifting toward justice and wellbeing.

With the groundwork of what and why established, the second section, "The Truth," deals with how to move to a higher level of consciousness. Chapter Six walks through how to assess your level of consciousness by becoming a witness observer. Using all our senses, we can understand our stresses and triggers and move toward a connected life. Chapter Seven offers examples of transforming practices that, if claimed as habit and daily rituals, can change us at the cellular level. Changing your practice will change you. Chapter Eight shows how mindfulness will allow doing to be replaced by being. Your calm will invite others to let go of their fear, too.

If you are embracing a life of mindful intention, you are not alone. Chapter Nine addresses the importance of utilizing sacred texts, teachers, coaches, friends, and supportive communities. Let them call you to a higher self and stay on track. The journey to higher consciousness is a spiritual journey, and it will also change your brain through neuroplasticity. Chapter Ten explains how to identify when our fight, flight, or freeze reaction isn't serving us, and how we can direct our attention to go instead to a place of calm where a higher transformative consciousness can be maintained.

Part Three, "The Light," takes a more in-depth look at **I am Interconnected** and **I am Infinite**. Chapter Eleven unfolds the second level where joy, intuition, ecstasy, creativity, and mysticism reside. Relationships improve. Toxicity evaporates, and our being invites others to a more beautiful place. Chapter Twelve presents the third level as holiness where the sense of self includes all that is. Your cells are in line with the cells of all creatures, balanced, and divine.

Finally, Part Four, "The World," sets higher consciousness loose to run free on earth. There are real relational and organizational benefits from living in a higher consciousness. Chapter Thirteen explores what happens when we become more present in relationships, listening as a witness in conversation, using authentic communication. Holes heal and our work together is more healthy and joyful. Your team works toward a goal positively. This chapter articulates how higher consciousness will make you into an effective leader at work and in your community. You will help your team feel safe, feel they belong, feel they matter, are heard, and are contributing. It will be contagious, spilling over to personal and professional lives.

Chapter Fourteen imagines what the world will look like if we move toward higher consciousness together. We are writing a new chapter and new history with more cooperative and effective relationships, business, and education systems. All aspects of life, from the arts to government, from economics to health, from culture to families, will reflect the shift toward peace.

The universe is calling us to embrace a higher consciousness, to mature into the new era with ease and joy. *Living From the Center Within* spans theory and practice in an accessible and exciting way. It utilizes sacred texts, real life stories, and science. Invitations to practice and reflection questions will help the reader internalize the material and know real transformation.

I am aware that I do not live everything proposed as possible when living in higher consciousness. On the journey, our alignment with the highest consciousness can be temporary and fleeting. Thus I can, at times, feel hypocritical about advocating for others to live at higher levels of consciousness when I do not live there continuously. However, my experience has taught me that each of us is a powerful catalyst for transformation. This knowing compels me to continue practicing. I, like my students and clients, am a work in progress.

Cultivating higher consciousness in myself and others delights me. I am grateful for the opportunities to write, teach, coach, and explore this passion. I invite you to join more deeply into this conversation so that together we may build our capacity to live at higher levels of consciousness. There are new resources, guided visualizations, class offerings, and blog postings on my website www.CenterWithin.com. Please be in touch. In your own circles I encourage you to connect and build the community of people living with intention and expanding our awareness. I invite each of us to support one another as we co-create who we are each becoming with love and compassion.

PART ONE

THE WAY: SEEING THE HOLES

CHAPTER 1

ASSESSING OUR PRESENT CONDITION

We each contribute to reconstructing a new inter-connected world by approaching our calling with a sense of wonder and curiosity.

What an amazing time to be on the planet. We are experiencing radical changes in the way we know and see ourselves and the world. Two decades ago, I got information from an encyclopedia, hand wrote letters, and only had a landline to talk on the telephone. I wrote directions on slips of paper. Now, in the age of the Internet, social media, and cell phones, information is available to me instantaneously. I can send a microloan to a woman farmer in Mali. I can read up on Reiki to relieve migraines. GPS directs me. I can request an Uber driver and use Yelp reviews in a new place. I have access to TED Talks, MIT courses, and the latest research on new scientific discoveries. I can read ancient wisdom teachings that were reserved for those living in monasteries.

Many rapid simultaneous changes are shifting our world-view, the perspective from which we see and interpret the world.

There are numerous leaps in understanding that are creating discontinuous gaps between what is and what came before. Paradigms, shared and accepted sets of assumptions, concepts, values, and beliefs that inform our view of reality are adjusting. Paradigms are being challenged and replaced by a new set of foundational ideas about reality that are profoundly different from those they are replacing. We are each being invited to co-create our personal, professional, and collective lives out of these new paradigms and expanding worldviews.

This shift also leads to more transparency. We know about a politician's affairs and a professional athlete's domestic violence. We can read about tax evasion and illegal activities previously hidden in offshore companies. We see large bands of garbage floating in our oceans. We are using body cameras on police officers, and drones in war zones. This intense increase of information accessibility is exciting and overwhelming.

New knowledge and changes are occurring in long-standing systems such as healthcare, government, education, and business. In health care, people have access to information and healers throughout the world. The western model treated illness with drugs and surgery. The integration of energy and holistic medicine is slowly transforming our focus towards prevention and the wellness of the whole person.

Non-government organizations (NGOs) are nonprofit organizations that engage in activities such as human rights, food and medical services, education, environmental protection, or economic development work that is defined in their mission statement. Previously this type of work was often done by governments, religions, or individual philanthropists. More and more communication, education, and fundraising is happening online through social media. Education can be received in part or totally from online schools at every level of learning. Global online educational projects support collaborative communication between students and teachers around the world.

In business, people lacking opportunities to build credit, gain employment, and acquire collateral are candidates for micro loans. Folks who were kept out of conventional financial lending opportunities can now become borrowers. These loans are empowering individuals, especially women and transforming entire communities through supporting entrepreneurship and alleviating poverty. Collectively, we are expanding and changing old ways of thinking and living. We are becoming global citizens.

Fundamental change provokes intense fear for some, causing grief and suffering. Uncertainty can be hard. It can evoke feelings of being overwhelmed or even paralyzed. Old systems are disintegrating, which is scary. Even if the systems were not serving us, the change can can be excruciating.

We have options. We can cling to old, dysfunctional worldviews, which could lead to our extinction. Or we can expand our perspective, create new models, and evolve into beings capable of greater love and collaboration. We can continue to use defensive and outdated thinking and behavior, which will only reinforce a sense of helplessness. Or we can become less fearful, less polarized, and choose instead to be more transparent, compassionate, interdependent, and solution-oriented. We can choose to see this as an epic moment in human history. We can create a new world where abundance, peace, cooperation, and sustainability are the norm.

It is important to assess our present condition and identify gaps and holes in our human condition. Parts of our environment are being abused and destroyed. There is injustice, unprecedented extremes of wealth and poverty, terrorism on a global scale, instability, a rapidly deteriorating biosphere, ecological disasters, record planetary population, garbage floating in our oceans, and unsustainable consumption. Violence streams into our eyes, ears, and hearts as we watch human beings abusing, exploiting, and murdering other human beings on our televisions, and technology screens.

How do we maximize growth and development in this time of shifting paradigms while some choose to desperately cling to old systems? We each can contribute to reconstructing a new, interconnected world. We write a new story about being human. We develop better education, healthcare, commerce, buildings, information exchange, energy sources, and media. We shift our political, economic, and cultural institutions. We form new systems to better serve humanity. How do you fit into these changes? Which paradigm shifts are you contributing to?

Each one of us is interconnected through a vast energy field. What we do, think, say, and feel changes this field. Quantum physicists show us how all matter is interrelated. They show how subatomic particles lack definitive physical properties and are defined only by the probabilities of being in different states. A particle exists in a suspended state, a sort of super-animation, until it is actually observed. Depending on the method of

area of the brain that is responsible for co
compassion. Learning to relax, reflect, st
have real effects on our wellbeing.
with our thoughts matters. These
are changing our perspective, g
new solutions for individua
from a completely new
As a transforma
changes in our u
technology, an
of my client
creativity
skills
re

insid

genetic information. Whetner we

produce different chemicals that impact our DNA. These che
icals can turn off and on parts of our DNA called genes, which can cause or prevent disease. Telomeres protect the ends of our DNA strands, acting like plastic tips at the end of shoelaces. Stress chemicals eat away at telomeres, literally shortening our lifespan by shortening the lifespan of the DNA.

We grow new brain cells and new brain cell connections every day. The part of our brain that grows is determined by the focus of our attention. If we choose to focus on trauma and drama, we grow the part of our brains responsible for survival, fight, and flight. If we are calm and non-reactive, we grow the

nplex reasoning and
ay calm, and empathize
earning to be intentional
ew insights into brain activity
ving us an opportunity to create
growth, development, and wellness
nderstanding.

onal coach, my clients and I discuss how
derstanding of interconnection, expanding
shifting paradigms in systems impact us. Many
s are visionaries with a desire to fully access their
, innovation, passion, and power. Together we practice
o deepen wisdom and compassion. We develop self-di-
ted plans to make the changes they desire in their lives. This
emerging new era in human history has a sense of urgency. It is time for each of us to pay attention to our deep longing and calling and to use our gifts, talents, and strengths to contribute in all areas of our lives.

Have you noticed the movers and shakers in their 20s? Ryan has been a friend of my daughter since high school, and we meet a few times a year to talk about the events of our unfolding lives. One topic sure to be discussed is Ryan's non-profit, Kibera Girls Soccer Academy Foundation (KGSA), which supports a school that provides free secondary education, artistic programming, and athletic opportunities to girls in the Kibera slum of Nairobi, Kenya. The NGO is a collaborative partnership. Ryan feels a connection to the girls in the school. He utilizes his passion and talents to usher in a new era of global citizens. His eyes and voice light up when he shares stories about enhancing the opportunities for girls in Kenya through education.

What excites you? Imagining how to transform nuclear waste into non-radioactive material? Implementing curriculum for children that addresses emotional, social, spiritual, and conversational intelligence? How about creating energy from a source that is efficient, accessible, and in harmony with all creatures? Do you have the ability to enhance healing or create art? We each contribute to reconstructing a new interconnected world by approaching our calling with a sense of wonder and curiosity. These new discoveries and solutions can fill humanity's holes.

An invitation from the 12th Century Sufi poet from Persia, Hafiz, translated by Daniel Ladinsky:

Now is the Time to Know

Now is the time to know
That all that you do is sacred.
Now, why not consider
A lasting truce with yourself and God?

Now is the time to understand
That all your ideas of right and wrong
Were just a child's training wheels
To be laid aside
When you can finally live
with veracity and love.

Now is the time for the world to know
That every thought and action is sacred.
This is the time
For you to compute the impossibility
That there is anything
But Grace.
Now is the season to know
That everything you do
Is Sacred.[1]

This book is an invitation to people interested in positively impacting who we are becoming. It is a map to discovering and living from our **Center Within**, that essential nature and ever-present Divine presence. It is a collection of wisdom learned through study, experiences, and contemplation. I have collected the process and tools described in this book through many years of healing, leading, coaching, and teaching. The information is not unique to me; the unfolding of my awareness offers one more voice in the choir of seekers and seers sharing their journeys, stories, and perspectives to this global dialogue of transformation.

As you read, expand your awareness, gather your attention, clarify your intention, and explore what it means to cultivate openings to higher consciousness and live from your **Center Within**. We already have what we need to make a shift to higher consciousness with ease, flow, and grace. The answer lies in applying both ancient wisdom and modern insights to

---

1. Daniel Ladinsky, "Now Is The Time to Know," *The Gift* (New York: Penguin, 1999), 18.

our present moment. This can lead to inner peace, balance, tolerance, harmony, vitality, and equanimity.

Invitation to Practice

- Take a deep breath in through your nose and out through your mouth. Feel your belly soften and expand. Repeat three times.

- Continue deep breathing. On your in-breath say the word "inspire" in your mind. Imagine fresh air and life-affirming ideas filling your lungs and permeating into each cell. Feel the freshness and lightness in your mind and body.

- On your out-breath, say the word "expire" in your mind. Imagine the release of ideas and beliefs that will not serve you as they leave each cell and flow out your lungs. Feel the spaciousness and vitality in your mind and body.

- In this relaxed condition, take a few moments for contemplation. Is there an area in your life that is ready for a change towards more ease and flow? Allow creative ideas and next steps to arise. What would this shift in your life ideally look like? Imagine this area of your life optimally benefiting you and all involved.

Take a few moments to capture your vision by drawing or writing about this shift in your life.

Let's co-create new stories about who we are becoming in our families, communities, and institutions both personally and collectively. Living full out and fearlessly is essential during this remarkable passage in humanity. As the ancient and ageless wisdom keepers tell us, we are the ones we have been waiting for.

Reflection

What are the issues in our changing world that you are the most passionate about? Why? How can you be a catalyst for transformation in these areas?

How do you cultivate a holistic and hopeful worldview within your circle of influence?

How do you positively engage with people and media that can drain your energy with negative thinking and messages?

How do you nurture relationships that foster mutual expansion?

How do you contribute to paradigm shifts in yourself? Your relationships? Your family? Your community? Your workplace? Our human family at large?

What excites you and makes your heart sing?

CHAPTER 2

EXPLORING NEW PARADIGMS

We have a choice to make: focus on what is ending or focus on what is beginning.

Why, during times of rapid growth, such as the extraordinary leap in human development occurring now, can it feel so disorientating? The transformational process is one of major change, which can feel stressful. When nature reaches a limitation, it innovates and transforms, evolving towards higher consciousness and more freedom. Since the beginning of life nearly four billion years ago, there has been a continuous movement towards complexity, connectivity, and higher levels of awareness. In the beginning, the planet finally cooled down so that the tiny basic fragments of matter were able to come together to form atoms. This was a quantum leap to a new level of substance. As cooling continued, atoms became molecules. Water emerged from the reaction of hydrogen and oxygen. It is a totally different material that bears no resemblance to the elements of the individual atoms.

As chemistry proceeded to become more and more complex, huge new compounds formed and joined with others in chemical reactions until some systems became so large and interdependent with many self-catalyzing reactions that groups of compounds began to reproduce and change. Life occurred, another quantum leap to a totally unpredictable advanced process. Life forms have transitioned from single cell, to multicellular, to vertebrates with central nervous systems, to mammals, to hominids, to Homo sapiens. The pace of this natural movement has been quickening in recent history. Each successive step happens faster than the last.

So what is shifting? Are we giving birth to new life? There are dynamic changes occurring in our communities, institutions, and families. We are collectively shifting within our hearts, minds, beliefs, and paradigms. We seem to be on the brink of another radical shift in our human life form. Each person has a choice: to focus on what is disintegrating or what is emerging. Depending on your perspective, it can appear to be either an ending or a beginning.

The process is similar to the birth of a baby. Recently, my grandson was born. After months of incremental change, drastic changes began for him just before birth. If my viewpoint were from inside of the womb, I'd see his birth as a nurturing environment disappearing: pressure and violent movements disturbing him, and light invading his safe, dark space. Death would seem imminent. Of course, my perspective was from the outside. I was experiencing joyful anticipation with my son, his wife, and our family, knowing he would be completely nourished, loved and cared for in a radically changed environment.

Think of this transformation on the planet as a "birth quake." It is a time of ending one era and beginning another. How you perceive this experience will impact how you feel about it. If you view the changes from where we have been, like the birth of a baby from inside the womb, all you see is how things used to be and how they are being destroyed or replaced by new ways.

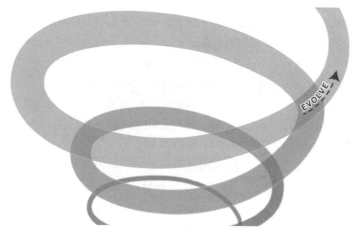

As I contemplate the transformation we are undergoing, an image of a spiral arises. Human beings have been traveling on a spiral of time through space. We are moving around the bend of a long gradual ascent, whipping around the outer edge of a sharp curve, which will move us towards another long gradual ascent at a higher level. Poised on the outside edge, we may hurl ourselves off the edge, or we may turn direction and remain evolving on the path of the spiral. Humanity is at a choice point of intense possibilities and opportunities, a transition that creates conditions for new perspectives and capacities to emerge.

Focusing on how things used to be may cause suffering or despair. Do you only look backwards? Do you long for the days when some people felt secure knowing they could work at the same company for their entire careers and feel assured they would have a pension in retirement? Do you resent the constant stream of news on war, hate crimes, and violence? Do you dwell on the negative feelings and fear?

Focusing on the future and rejecting the past is also limiting. To rebel and revolt against what has been can be destructive and does not promote positive change and expanding awareness. Do you complain about what is wrong and give your time and attention to being in opposition to what is occurring? Do you discard the wisdom of past teachings and established norms and culture?

Another option is to decide to open the lens of perception and embrace change, transcending and including as we move into higher levels of complexity. Rather than causing a sense of constriction, you may notice your worldview expanding. In addition, this perspective increases the likelihood of feeling ease, calmness, and clarity. Do you embrace opportunities to learn about new ideas and cultures? Do you continue developing your gifts and talents and seek new challenges? Do you apply your passions and expertise in service to new solutions?

When we relax and trust the process of the birthquake occurring in humanity as a natural progression of development, we open our imagination to create and innovate. By doing this, we are more capable of intentionally participating in impacting who we are becoming as we transition into this new era of being human. This process is the process of co-creating a new paradigm. We focus on envisioning a future that supports the highest good for all beings. We give our allegiance to the dawning of what is beginning.

What could this new era look like for us personally and collectively? Following is a list of possible qualities of the eras, which are both ending and beginning to start our conversation. They could pertain to us personally, interpersonally, professionally or collectively. We can see these qualities shifting in our communities and society at large. We know them in our inner beliefs, thoughts, and hearts. Noticing them is our first step. Once we can recognize when our choices are based in worry or tightness, we can choose to step back, reflect, and evaluate if our fears are coming from what is actually occurring or an outdated belief or habitual response. We can actively intend to create our inner and outer experiences with more trust and openness.

Can you get a sense of the constriction of some of the qualities of the old era crumbling? Can you feel the expansion of the possible qualities of a new era? Let's visualize our future together.

Imagine a bridge connecting the old era to the new era. Each person is free to cross the bridge into the new era at his or her own pace, in his or her own way. The force of change is so powerful that complacency is not an option. This shift is felt and seen by all. Each person's response to changes are chosen by their free will and preferences. It is not up to us to impose our pace of change or perspective on others. We must live our lives not focused on the fear of what is falling apart, but be an example by embracing what is emerging.

Qualities of the Old Era	Qualities of the New Era
Depletion	Sustainability
Secrecy	Transparency
Citizens with borders	Global/Universal citizens
Hidden information	Shared information
Exclusivity	Inclusivity
Self-serving	Mutually beneficial
Despising differences	Honoring diversity
Separation	Interconnectedness
Blame	Responsibility
Win-Lose strategies	Win-Win strategies
Alienate	Collaborate
External locus of power and responsibility	Internal locus of power and responsibility
Scarcity	Abundance
Deconstruction	Reconstruction
Polarization	Common ground
Greed	Compassion
Antagonism	Solidarity
Violence	Peace
Entitlement	Mutual accountability
Agitation	Equanimity
Dominance	Freedom
Break down	Break through
Discrimination	Equality
Communication requiring time and space	Instantaneous communication

Some people are kicking and screaming on the path leading to the bridge of transformation and may be warning us to resist change. Paradigm-busting insights and ideas have historically met with fervent opposition. In the shifting paradigm of medicine, health and wellness for instance, there is strong opposition by some entrenched allopathic practitioners towards energy, integrative, or holistic medical practices. Conventional providers use terms like hoax, dangerous, invalid, and unscientific to describe these treatments. Some refuse to accept the new paradigms and cling to the old mechanistic model of the body. Each of us embrace advancing knowledge and mindsets at our own pace. We are invited to release judgment, and allow and trust the timing of the process.

Others are integrating new ways of being and knowing while remaining in the current structures of institutions and organizations. Building the bridge to our new dimension within established systems and structures is valuable. Continuing on our shifting medical practice example, hospital systems are creating wellness centers, health coaching programs and meditation classes. Inside some health care facilities, clinicians are offering guided imagery, healing touch, acupuncture and aromatherapy. It requires patience and passion to stay in old era systems and incorporate new era changes.

Invitation to Practice

- Find a quiet place to relax and close your eyes. Take a few deep breaths.

- To facilitate relaxing deeply, I invite you to focus on slowly tensing and then relaxing adjoining muscle groups in your body progressing from your feet to your head. Start by tensing and relaxing the muscles in your toes and feet for at least 5 seconds and then relax for 5-30 seconds. Repeat with a new muscle group moving up your lower leg, then upper legs, and repeat in small sections up your body until you reach your head. Continue breathing deeply.

- Once complete and you are deeply relaxed, pick one quality of the new era you would like to cultivate in your life. Imagine, see, and contemplate this attribute and feel it expand in your awareness. How would cultivating this quality create changes in your own life? How would it contribute to shifting into the new era?

Take a few minutes to record your insights with words or drawings.

There are cutting edge researchers, teachers, mystics, and visionaries exploring and creating in this new frontier of being human. As has been true throughout human history, often the compelling evidence of new wisdom and insights being discovered challenges conventional ideas. Those creating in new paradigms and systems are often rejected by their peers and the mainstream. In the medical models example, we are seeing entirely new fields of practice in neuroscience, food as medicine, energy, and spiritual healing. These incorporate a deeper understanding of the field that connects all life and the interdependence of the mind, body and spirit. They focus on balance and prevention and are radically changing our old ideas of what is best for fighting disease and promoting health.

In my own life, I have traveled the bridge of transformation through several career changes. My last full-time work as an employee was working for a national health care company managing four locations which served twelve states. During the ten years I worked there, I created a number of leadership and professional development programs that included mutual accountability, win-win strategies, empathy, and compassion. We honored diversity in strengths, perspectives, and talents, as well as cultures and backgrounds. My division was highly successful in both human and financial performance. I worked with like-minded change agents throughout the organization to create new era systems in an old era organization. We developed and implemented new ways of providing home health care and new ways of cultivating leaders.

My consulting business offering personal, interpersonal, and organizational coaching was growing, and I took the leap and began self-employment full time. There were a number of friends and family who adamantly attempted to talk me out of that decision. What was I thinking leaving a six-figure income job for no security and no guaranteed work? How can the potential freedom, creativity, innovation, and collaborative opportunities be worth the loss of comfort in a set hierarchy, good retirement benefits, and the support of an established boss and organization? Some who could not tolerate my risk taking and allegiance to that which makes my heart sing rejected me.

Yes, there were times when the transitions felt overwhelming or challenging. I have walked to the bridge leading me to the next step of my truth with resistance at times. I have crossed the bridge into a new era in my own life and felt the anxiety of being in unfamiliar territory. Where do I find the best health insurance for self-employed individuals? Do I offer coaching in a home office? If not, where do I find an affordable and supportive space? How do I attract clients and projects that nurture and sustain me? How do I get started on a website and social media platforms? There have been many opportunities to practice trusting the process, having clear intention and keeping my attention in the present moment.

Having been a full-time consultant for many years now, the work that has come to me is in alignment with what makes my heart sing. The courses I teach at the Center for Spirituality & Healing at the University of Minnesota nurture and open my heart. They also engage and challenge both my logical, analytical left brain and my holistic, intuitive right brain. I have created new courses that incorporate ancient ageless wisdom teachings, mindfulness practices, and discoveries in mind-body science. I have become more transparent, humble, inclusive, and innovative. This opportunity provides amazing student interactions as well as continual learning through colleagues and other faculty.

My private coaching business allows me to be with individuals and organizations that are becoming more authentic and courageous every day. We explore their growing edges and release outdated and limiting beliefs while cultivating and expanding their inner passions and talents. My clients teach me compassion, tolerance, and equanimity. In working with leaders and organizations, we continue to deepen skills in collaborating, finding common ground, and honoring diversity.

The workshops I develop and offer continue to bring new information from research, life experience, and my own inner exploration into expression. Creating them requires me to get clear and articulate in sharing information. The participants continuously encourage me to find ways to engage in this discussion of new era creation as a local and global citizen. These opportunities also bring up my fears and resistance. I have been invited to create connection, community, and workshops through new technology that intimidates and scares me. I have found amazing resources and support for the components of my work that I find difficult, and focus my attention and intention on my natural abilities and strengths.

For me, leaving my full-time steady income corporate job to pursue consulting has ushered me into the new era. You too can make small choices that move you into further alignment with what makes your heart sing. You too can create a life that you love. We are each invited to fully own our role as a visionary co-creating our new era. Lao Tzu, a 6th Century BCE Chinese philosopher and author of the Tao-Te Ching, encourages us to do the same:

There is no need
to run outside
for better seeing,
Nor to peer from a window.
Rather abide at the center of your being;
for the more you leave it, the less you learn.
Search your heart
and see.
If he is wise who takes each turn:
the way to do
is to be.[2]

Reflection

Which activities, thoughts, beliefs, and paradigms do you need to release to move forward into this new world?

Which activities, thoughts, beliefs, and paradigms expand your human capacity, creativity, and awareness and lend support for this emerging world of abundance?

How do the new systems emerging impact your life?

What vision do you hold for our future as human beings on this home called Earth?

---

2.   Lau Tzu, #47 from *The Way of Life According to Lao-Tzu* edited by Witter Bynner (New Tork: Perigree, 1986), 75. See credit, legal page iv.

CHAPTER 3

SHIFTING PERSPECTIVE

As we embody higher levels of consciousness, our capacity to co-create who we are becoming personally, interpersonally, organizationally, in our families, communities, institutions, and globally is enhanced.

What does all that have to do with co-creating and improving humanity? Let's start with exploring consciousness. I understand consciousness to be a vast interconnected field of which everything is a part. It is the large unified energy field that we know connects everything, seen and unseen, throughout the cosmos. This field contains intelligence and provides connectivity for instantaneous communication. It conducts the energy of the observer to change a particle to a waveform seen in quantum physics. I imagine consciousness as a large sea that includes all that is. Like a vast sea, waves continue to form and return to the water. Each wave has a beginning, middle, and end, yet is not separate from sea itself. The water in the sea is continuously connected while it is shifting. Similarly, the changing manifest world is constantly informed by the sea of consciousness.

Our individual awareness dictates how much of this sea we can sense. Awareness is the state or ability to perceive, know, realize, and make meaning of our experience. As we expand our awareness, we increase our capacity to experience more levels of this very expansive sea or field of consciousness. As our perception opens wider, our understanding of the interconnected nature of the field deepens. This in turn updates, expands, and shifts our paradigms and worldviews.

As I contemplate levels of consciousness and my desire to communicate it clearly, the picture that comes to me is a cell in the human body. Imagine you are looking at a cell through a microscope with very high magnification that can bring into focus the smallest particles we can see. You would observe tiny particles at a quantum level such as quarks, leptons, and bosons, which are the essential building blocks of the cell. At the quantum level, one particle can exist in two different places at the same time. Two particles can be entangled and when one changes its state, the other will do so immediately, acting faster than the speed of light. Particles can also tunnel through seemingly solid objects, like a ghost passing through a wall. These barriers are impenetrable to larger objects.

As you change the power of your microscope lens and widen your focus, you notice these particles combine to form protons, electrons, and neutrons, which are components of an atom. Like the quantum level, the atomic level of the cell has unique properties, governing principles and functions. Protons and neutrons are in the center of an atom, making up the nucleus. Electrons surround the nucleus. Protons have a positive charge, electrons have a negative charge. All particles at the quantum and atomic levels are contained in the exact same time and space.

If we continue to widen the focus of our microscope lens, we notice atoms combine to form molecules. Like the quantum and atomic levels, the molecular level has unique governing principles and functions. Molecules are made of a fixed numbers of atoms joined together by bonds and can be gases, liquids, or solids. The molecules in turn create various parts of the cell such as a cell wall, lysosomes, ribosomes, and mitochondria. The quantum, atomic, and molecular levels concurrently exist in the same space and time. What you see is determined by your level of focus.

Continuing to broaden our lens, we see the molecules that make up the cell itself. If we don't stop there, and continue widening our view, we notice this cell is part of an organ in the body. The organ is part of the entire body, which is part of the body of living beings on Earth, which is part of our solar system, which is part of our galaxy, which is part of the universe, which is part of multiple universes. The structures function separately with different principles at each plane of magnification. Simultaneously each level exists in the same time and space with ongoing interactions and defined relationships with all forms at every dimension.

How does this metaphor extend to levels of consciousness? There are many ideas and models for levels of consciousness. They have been described by psychologists, scientists, quantum physicist, mystics, philosophers, healers, educators, and evolution-of-consciousness theorists. You can learn more about other models of consciousness through resources listed in the resource section. Through my years of study, life experiences, client work, and insights discovered through inner exploration, I have developed a model that is simplified into three levels of consciousness.

The levels of consciousness are:

- **I am Individual.** This is the first stage of human development. Here our self-identification is limited to our own bodies, thoughts, emotions, personal stories, and experiences; everyone and everything else is not self.

- **I am Interconnected.** This is the second stage of human development. Here our perception shifts to realize self as an individual who is interconnected. We recognize our experience is directly and continuously affected by and connected to what is occurring outside of our personal bodies, emotions, and thoughts.

- **I am Infinite.** This is the third stage of human development. Here, self and other disappear into one, and awareness is all that exists. We experience all form having a beginning, middle and end and arising from pure awareness.

Each expanded level of consciousness encompasses the previous level, just like a whole cell contains the quantum, atomic, and molecular level. Generally, as a human develops, **I am Individual** is our initial experience of self. We know ourselves as separated from everyone and everything else. As we expand our viewpoint to a larger perspective like widening our focus through the microscope lens, **I am Interconnected** emerges into our awareness. In addition to seeing ourselves as an individual, we simultaneously recognize ourselves as part of the interconnected field of consciousness. If we continue to expand awareness, we come to know ourselves not only as an individual and as interconnected in the sea of consciousness, but also as **I am Infinite.** From this point of view, we realize we ultimately are the entire vast field of consciousness itself. We recognize the uniqueness, whether a particle or person, and concurrently realize they are not separate from the whole.

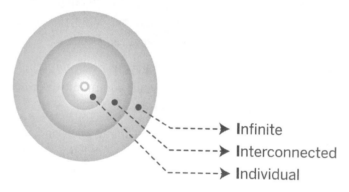

Embodying higher levels of consciousness is essential for us to co-create new solutions, structures, and paradigms. Fortunately, it is a natural human tendency to move toward ever-expanding levels of consciousness. We continuously evolve towards progressively greater knowledge, complexity, and capacity while embracing our previous level of development. We transcend earlier limitations and realize more profound understanding. This shift is accompanied by new priorities,

Invitation to Practice

- Find a few minutes to deeply relax. Take a few cleansing breaths and feel your belly soften while it rises and falls.

- Imagine you are sitting in a peaceful place. Maybe it was a place you visited on vacation. Maybe a favorite place in your home. Allow yourself to remember the sights, sounds, smells, tastes, and feel of this place. Adjust your experience in your mind, creating the perfect relaxing place for this moment. Allow this image to fade as the sense of deep peace remains.

- Visualize a microscope shifting focus from your cells to your organs to your body to your community. Who or what do you feel connected to?

- Imagine your point of view continuing to expand. You can now visualize the entire planet with her land, seas, winds, animals, and plants. What connection do you see, sense, know, or experience?

- Return your attention to your breath. When and where do you encounter moments of deepest connection in your life?

- Take a few minutes to feel your gratitude for these connections and, if you like, record your experience.

resources and abilities. In my experience, as we embody higher levels of consciousness, our capacity to co-create who we are becoming personally, interpersonally, organizationally, in our families, communities, institutions, and globally is enhanced.

Reflection

When have you felt isolated and disconnected from others? What is your experience in your body, thoughts and emotions?

When have you been in nature and felt the deep connection to the land, wind, sun or water? How did it feel in your body? What were your emotions? Did you observe any thoughts?

When have you noticed a connection to someone else not in your physical presence? How did you know you were connected?

What are the feelings in your body, heart, and mind when you relax into ease, flow, and joy?

CHAPTER FOUR

EMBODYING CONSCIOUSNESS

Freeing our attention and clarifying our intention,
our daily lives becomes more congruent, integrated,
authentic, and coherent.

How are **I am Individual, I am Interconnected,** and **I am Infinite** embodied in everyday living? Let's take a closer look. We understand that in every human being, all levels of consciousness exist simultaneously and continuously. Unless we are fully developed or realized, we do not generally have access at will to all levels. Although the progression of expanding our perspective is not linear, it often follows a common path of unfolding in our awareness.

For most people, initially we know ourselves as **I am Individual.** We experience a world of duality. The locus of identity is on personal emotions, thoughts, impulses, images, and sensations contained in our own body and separate from everything else. We are the subject of our experience. Because of this, we often experience a sense of vigilance and need to protect ourselves. It can be difficult to feel satisfied and complete. There is often an underlying sense of fear and lack. Often our attention is not in the present moment and wanders to worry about the future or ruminates on the past, sometimes without even noticing.

At the most underdeveloped perspective in **I am Individual**, we can believe that anyone who is not like us, who does not share the same beliefs, history, or skin color as us, is dangerous.

With the justification that these differences in others are threatening, people throughout history with this self-centered focus have oppressed and killed other human beings. These immature viewpoints can prevail in social institutions, such as religious groups or political parties as well. It is time for us as a global family to transcend this fear-based and violent behavior.

As we develop at this level of consciousness, we work to gain possessions, status, or approval. There is often an inner sense of insufficiencies in self-love or self-worth. Holes can present themselves as limiting beliefs and negative self-talk. As we continue to progress we move towards balance and maturity. We expand intelligences such as emotional, physical, social, intellectual, relational, and financial. These skills increase our inner sense of satisfaction and "fill in our holes" or sense of lack. We develop towards an inner sense of wholeness.

In my life, these holes took the form of giving both to my family and at work until I was depleted. There was an underlying sense that I had to do more to prove myself and get ahead. I was raised in a family system where we were long on duty and responsibility and short on compliments and encouragement. I remember being told, "Don't get too big for your britches," encouraging me to play small.

Through my own suffering and exhaustion I learned to meditate, went on retreats, found friends who lived their passions, learned and practiced balance, reduced my stress, and sang more. My holes healed. I released the messages I had internalized that were not true, and created new beliefs and habits that nurtured me back to wholeness. I began to make small healthy choices that created a life of love.

As we feel more harmony and calm inside our bodies, emotions, and thoughts, this condition informs the worldview we use to see each other. The other out there no longer feels so threatening, and we begin to cultivate tolerance. Judgment diminishes. As we move towards fulfillment at the **I am Individual** level of consciousness, our focus on doing can lead us to become productive and contributing citizens. We have meaningful relationships, and feelings of purpose, self-confidence, and passion. The holes created by lack of self-worth and self-love heal. We begin feeling complete and whole. Humanity would be radically transformed and improved if every person fully embodied this level of consciousness.

CONSCIOUSNESS LEVEL	FOCUS
Individual	Healing Holes
Interconnected	Becoming Whole
Infinite	Being Holy

When identification expands to **I am Interconnected**, we realize that inner experiences of thoughts, feelings, and body sensations are often connected to occurrences outside of our personal selves. We remain the subject of our experiences but recognize the connection to the objects we perceive. For example, we notice changes in our bodies, when it tightens up and when it relaxes, depending upon our surroundings. We pay more attention to our impulses, and often make choices based on a quiet thought or knowing. With the inner stillness that resides as our baseline experience most of the time, we become increasingly aware of the connections that are always present. This creates the conditions for us to more readily notice subtle energy such as intuition, synchronicity, or information that comes to us in a sleeping or day dream. Here is a story reported by a client:

> My mother began a long, slow, painful demise into Alzheimer's disease in her 80s. As her brain began to unravel, I came to dread my weekly visits to her, it was just so painful to watch. She had been a harsh and critical woman and my relationship with her as an adult had been guarded. After she passed, even though it seemed a great relief, I struggled with grief. One night she "came to me" in a dream, and took me on a drive down a country road. In the dream, as we drove over the crest of a hill, we came upon the most beautiful field of white and purple flowers, and I realized that she was just showing me where she was now. I woke out of sound sleep, sobbing. After some time, I fell back asleep, and curiously into the same dream with her. This time, I asked her if I still needed to come visit her (during her demise), and she tenderly leaned over me, cupped my face in her hands. She was instantly transformed into the younger mom I knew and lovingly said "of course not." Once again, I woke out of a sound sleep, sobbing. Only afterward did I come to realize that this dream was more

"real" than most of the reality I was experiencing daily. I have never looked at life the same way since.

Another shift at this level of consciousness is understanding and experiencing paradox. Discernment replaces impulsive judgment. People, events, and thoughts are no longer viewed as being so clear-cut, always right or always wrong. We recognize them more on a continuum that is ever-shifting and changing. Each person, event, or thought has a beginning, middle and end. Our truths can appear to be contradictory on the surface. An example of a paradox holding multiple truths for a person at **I am Interconnected** level of consciousness might be the experience of having cancer. It can be the worst and best event in a person's life. We are no longer trapped in the constant, often previously unnoticed process of measuring, labeling, and comparing. We also come to see the cancer as a consequence of some unknown processes or activity that push us to question, "Why?" We are able to be in the fullness and complexity of the experience as a whole.

When this quantum leap in perspective occurs, we also increase our awareness of inspirations, revelations, and innovations. We begin to feel love not limited to our personal circle of friends and family, but expanding to include humanity at large. We tap into feeling causeless joy, not just prompted by an inner or outer personal event. Our worldview changes. Now we know and see ourselves as part of the sea of consciousness rather than separate from it. Duality still exists; there is still a separate "me" as a subject, perceiving the other as an object, but we are undeniably connected to all that is.

One client was struggling to find a job after graduating from college. He was ambiguous about joining his family on a vacation to Florida as he felt he should stay home and spend the time job hunting. He needed to decrease his mounting anxiety and relax and decided on the vacation. He set an intention to add focus, clarity, and ease to his job search. While driving down to Florida, he passed a car with the license plate with the word Brandon on it. Later that evening he was served by a waiter named Brandon. The next morning he received a text message from his friend Brandon letting him know they had an opening at his company and wondered if he had found a job. He interviewed when he returned and started his new job one week later.

When we live as **I am Interconnected,** we are often creative, fresh, alive, and prolific. A person living at this level of consciousness can live as a sage, mystic, artist, teacher, inventor, or healer. It is a level marked by tolerance, unity, trust, energy awareness, peacemaking, joy, ease, fearlessness, and intuition. Our primary sense of self is being whole and belonging to the sea of all beings in the field of consciousness. We feel complete, at peace, and trust that we are enough and have enough. We know we are worthy and loveable.

Einstein calls us to the wholeness of **I am Interconnected**:

A human being is part of the whole, called by "Universe"; a part limited in time and space. We experience ourselves, our thoughts and feelings, as something separated from the rest, a kind of optical delusion of our consciousness. This delusion is a kind of prison for us, restricting us to our personal desires and to affection for a few persons nearest to us. Our task must be to free ourselves from this prison by widening our circle of compassion to embrace all living creatures and the whole of nature in its beauty.[3]

Another quantum leap in perspective occurs when we experience ourselves as **I am Infinite** and subject and object merge into one identity. The perception that I am the subject experiencing the world and everything in it as the object disappears. What remains is pure awareness. We experience form (anything that has a beginning, middle, and end) in the world as shifting and changing moment to moment, like waves arising from the ocean. Yet, our primary identity becomes the entire field of consciousness which remains unchanging like the ocean itself.

Embodying **I am Infinite** level of consciousness may be familiar if you have been completely absorbed in an activity such as gardening or running where there is just one; not even a doer and the doing or seer and seeing. You lose yourself in the experience while remaining the person you are. This may also be perceived during deep dreamless sleep or love making where there is no awareness of where "I" ends and "my beloved" begins.

Psychiatrist David Hawkins eloquently describes this passage into **I am Infinite**:

> Desire for existence itself must be surrendered. Only when this is done may one finally move beyond allness or nothingness, beyond existence or non-existence. This culmination of the inner work is the most difficult phase, the ultimate watershed, where one is starkly aware that the illusion of existence one transcends here is irrecoverable. There's no

---

3. Quoted in Larry Dossey, *The Science of Premonitions: How Knowing the Future Can Help Us Avoid Danger* (New York: Penguin Group, 2010).

returning from this step and this specter of irreversibility makes this last barrier appear the most formidable choice of all. But, in fact, in this final apocalypse of the self, the dissolution of the sole remaining duality, that of existence and non-existence, identity itself, dissolves in universal divinity, and no individual consciousness is left to choose. The last step, then, is taken by God alone.[4]

The process of human development towards realizing higher levels of consciousness is not linear. Most of us live our day-to-day life primarily at one stage or level of consciousness. As we develop, we generally do not fully embody one level before taking a quantum leap into the next stage. In any given moment, we can have fleeting experiences at a much higher level. We may have what feels like a breakthrough experience that is a temporary state of consciousness higher than our ordinary reality. In fact, it is through these momentary experiences of access to larger views of the sea of consciousness that we learn how to move our attention from one level to the next. We move back and forth. The goal is to maintain as high a level of consciousness as possible in any given present moment: to remember we are Divine spirits having a human experience.

The edges of who and what we know ourselves to be expands gradually or radically through our experiences. Occasionally an event can expand our awareness very quickly. This is often an experience so outside of our ordinary understanding and paradigm that it stretches us beyond our familiar comfortable

---

4.   David Hawkins, *Power vs. Force: The Hidden Determinants of Human Behavior* (Carlsbad: Hay House, 2002), 24.

size, inviting us to question the limits of our current reality or viewpoint.

A client's entire worldview changed when he experienced a visit from his father. Receiving news that his father was near death, he got on an airplane to travel to his father's bedside. During the flight, he felt his father's presence. Upon arrival, he learned his father had passed at the time he felt his father's spirit visit him on the plane. His understanding of his ability to feel a presence that was no longer limited to a human body changed radically. Previously he had heard these experiences were possible. Once it was his own lived experience, he began a deeper quest into cultivating higher consciousness in his life. Over the years, he has become attuned to more subtle energy and ways of knowing. He has become what I would call an everyday mystic.

I had an experience when I was a child in church listening to a reading from the book of Psalms that forever changed my perception of the here and now. The passage spoke about the keys to the kingdom of heaven being contained in the Wisdom of Solomon. In that moment it felt like a portal opened, and I was in Solomon's temple. I heard people speaking a language I did not recognize. I could smell food cooking in open fire pits. I had an undeniable feeling I had been there before. It was not a daydream or thought, but a visceral lived experience.

This has led to a lifetime inquiry into the wisdom teachings of many traditions, including Solomon. Throughout my life I have had more encounters with the teachings and Wisdom of Solomon, which have guided me in unexpected and miraculous ways. While at a convention in Philadelphia, I went sightseeing one afternoon and happened upon the Masonic Temple. I remember standing in the lobby fascinated to learn about our founding fathers' involvement in an organization I knew almost nothing about. I came upon a small-scale replica of the temple of Solomon. To my amazement it was identical to the one I had visited as a child. More recently, after a large transition in my life, I was searching for a new place to live. With my children off to college, I would be living alone for the first time in years. I felt led to an amazing six condo building in a fabulous neighborhood in my city and bought it two days later. It was a converted 1899 Masonic Temple. During my years of living there I felt protected and nurtured.

The circumstance generating this type of internal realization or shift could be a book we read, a conversation we have, a relationship we begin or end, a workshop we attend, a new job, a walk in the woods, a dream, a physical or mental health change, or travel. There are many forms of meditation, which is a practice designed to bring all of our attention into the present moment, that can cultivate an awareness of and opening to a larger view of the sea of consciousness. We can experience this expansion in many ways such as an insight, release of energy, spaciousness in awareness, or a strong emotion.

Imagine blowing up a balloon. Each experience that expands access to higher consciousness is like adding air to the inside of a balloon. The balloon stretches in size with each new breath as the balloon gets tauter.

It may take time to integrate and adjust to this larger way of being and thinking in the world, and sometimes we revert to our

Invitation to Practice

- Find a few minutes to relax. Take a few deep breaths in through your nose and out through your mouth.

- Feel the energy of the earth rising through your feet and up your body. You are fully grounded and supported.

- Remember a time when you had an experience that was very real to you and seemed like a miracle and extraordinary. How did you know it was authentic? What impact did it have on your mind, body and emotions? How did it change your worldview or beliefs?

- Set your intention to notice information and knowing that presents itself to you that you "get" by perceiving beyond your 5 senses. Allow yourself to be curious and playful. Pay close attention to what arises in your awareness over the next few days. You can document your insights through journaling or engaging in the arts.

old patterns, habits and point of view. Just like the balloon blowing up, there is resistance as new air enters. It can feel like there is a force pushing back, trying to keep us small.

This resistance can feel like procrastination, fear of being seen, wounds, pain, or frustrations. We can stumble upon beliefs and limiting self-talk saying, "It needs to be hard" or, "It's not worthwhile" or, "I don't deserve to be too big." This growth can kick up buried messages that we are unlovable or unworthy and attempt to squeeze our expanding self back down to size. The remedy to this self-sabotaging is to give our allegiance to that which expands us and trust the natural process of our own and all human development.

Deep into writing this book, I had an experience of not having or being enough. I decided to ask for assistance in supporting the completion of this book through a crowd sourcing fundraising process called Kickstarter. While creating the campaign, I could feel my resistance. What if nobody contributed? I would be humiliated and feel foolish. As I launched the Kickstarter campaign and began more actively asking for backing, the worry increased. Memories of times I had not experienced encouragement and felt sabotaged came flashing back.

A few days after the campaign launched, I headed up to the cabin on a beautiful peaceful lake in northern Wisconsin. While creating Kickstarter email requests to friends and family one morning, I became dizzy and nauseated. I vomited and had diarrhea for 6 hours straight. I moved from the bed to the couch, staying close to the bathroom. My partner graciously checked in on me. He made some fabulous broth, and eventually it stayed down and I began to recover. The force of clearing in my body, emotions, and thoughts of times I had previously felt a need to stay small and protect myself was stunning. The process of writing this book has demanded more transparency, vulnerability and honesty than I had anticipated.

Healing the holes inside ourselves can be painful and frustrating. Developing our perceptive sensitivity to subtle energies and realities can come with second-guessing and confusion. The rewards of higher consciousness are worth it. We become more peaceful, trusting, and confident. We have the freedom to choose our responses calmly and compassionately. We have greater access to our creativity and inspiration.

As we continue to heal, we free our attention and clarify our intention. The boundaries and limits that kept us small eventually give way and we expand permanently to a new and larger capacity. Our daily life becomes more congruent, integrated, authentic, and coherent. We experience more joy, ease, and flow. This process of experiencing higher states of consciousness happens again and again, sometimes gradually and sometimes suddenly, until we stretch back and forth enough to comfortably remain in our expanded perspective at a radical new higher stage of consciousness. We become more capable of intentionally participating in impacting who we are becoming as we transition into this new era of being human.

Reflection

What event or events have assisted in expanding your awareness to higher levels of consciousness in your life?

What limiting beliefs, values, stories, thoughts, and habits do you bump up against as you expand into higher levels of consciousness?

Have you had a change in a long-standing belief, idea, or thought? What prompted this change in your viewpoint?

Have you experienced yourself as **I am Infinite**, where there was only pure awareness and no sense of separation or differentiation at all?

How do you gain access to higher levels of consciousness in your own experience?

CHAPTER FIVE

ACCEPTING THE INVITATION

*Living as the full expression of our true nature from our **Center Within** is a treasured gift to all beings.*

How does embodying higher levels of consciousness help us co-create a new world? One way we co-create is through service. The level of service we can provide is directly related to our level of consciousness. If we live in **I am Individual** consciousness, we can feel alienated and only trust our self. We experience others as separate and categorized, and there is ongoing judgment of each person relative to our own perceived status. There is an underlying belief in scarcity, a sense that any help we give each other must come from a finite pot of resources. For example, I have a fish and you are hungry. Living with a limiting viewpoint, my only choices appear to be keeping my fish and eating it, giving my fish to you and being hungry, or splitting the fish leaving both of us semi-satisfied.

Service from people living in **I am Individual**, whether in our own homes, at work, or on a volunteer project, can come from a desire for personal gain or have strings attached. There can even be a sense of debt owed by the receiver to the giver, or a belief by the giver that he or she is entitled to impose his or her views on the receiver.

Groups are made up of individuals at various stages of development. The group or system itself has its own level of consciousness. It is possible for a group to behave at immature levels while the members individually can live at higher levels. Institutions, whether political, economic, or cultural can also operate and co-create at this lower level of consciousness. Groups, formal or informal, go through stages of development just like individuals. We see this in organizations, families, and communities as well.

During 2008, 2010, and 2016, Haiti experienced multiple natural disasters. As I followed updates on the disaster relief efforts, I was disappointed to read about leaders and agencies vying for status. They competed for recognition and resources, duplicated one another's efforts, and generally got in one another's way. Because they could not work together, they compounded the situation of utter chaos. There was a focus on personal gain for the organizations rather than on collaborative service.

In 2010, ten American missionaries were charged with criminal conspiracy and kidnapping because they attempted to take thirty-three Haitian children across the border into the Dominican Republic without proper documentation. The missionaries said they were going to house the children in a converted hotel in the Dominican Republic and later move them to an orphanage they were building. However, any Haitian child needs government approval to leave the country, and the group acknowledged that the children had no passports. The Americans also claimed they were just trying to help the children leave the earthquake-stricken country. The missionaries were acting from **I am Individual.** They believed they knew what was best for these children. Their judgment and action disregarded the laws that govern the community they were serving. When we offer assistance while imposing our own preferences and viewpoints, our service is diminished. What we co-create through service at this level of consciousness is generally limited.

In **I am Interconnected** consciousness, we have wider access to the sea of consciousness and the connections it contains when we serve. We all have the innate capacity to join the work for the whole while embodying our own life purpose. When we are living in **I am Interconnected,** our beliefs move from scarcity in lower consciousness to abundance; we realize there is more than enough for everyone if we contribute what makes our heart sing from our essence and authenticity. Here, when we set an intention to create solutions, we may notice insight in something we read, in our dreams, or in our conversations. Innovation and creativity arise in ordinary and extraordinary ways.

We attune to our unique talents and gifts. We offer our service when an opportunity presents itself that feels expansive and aligns with our natural capacities. Picture a murmuration of starlings. Each bird joins the flock and out of the seeming chaos of flight, gorgeous, geometric patterns coalesce. They twist and turn and change direction at a moment's notice. When we operate at **I am Interconnected**, we come together and focus on a common cause. Initially it can feel like turmoil or upheaval. We pay attention and are ready to transform in an instant as we respond to each other and the situation with grace and beauty. We are poised to find the perfect group of people with complementary abilities, and produce a mutually beneficial energy exchange of resources such as time, ideas, skill, and money.

Our aim is to infuse wisdom and compassion into the institutions of our culture. We pursue transforming our schools, governance, health care systems, environment, and social policies. We feel a universal responsibility for all. Service becomes a sacred act and contains radical possibilities for new solutions and manifestations.

The timeless wisdom of Teilhard de Chardin invites us to weave expanding self-awareness and contributing in the world into our lives:

> The life of each one of us is, as it were, woven of those two threads: the thread of inward development, through which our ideas and affections and our human and spiritual attitudes are gradually formed; and the thread of outward success by which we always find ourselves at the exact point where the whole sum of the forces of the universe meet together to work in us as the effect which God desires.[5]

An example of service living as **I am Interconnected** is Einstein's experience of making discoveries. He describes how during dreaming and meditating, understandings of the nature of the universe arose as a "knowing" fully formed. When

---

5. Teilhard de Chardin, *The Divine Milieu: An Essay on the Interior Life*, (New York: Harper Torchbooks, 1957), 79.

summarizing the general theory of relativity, he stated that time, space and gravitation have no separate existence from matter. They are all contained in a single connected entity. What a wonderful description of the sea of consciousness. Mozart reports the same process, hearing entire orchestral arrangements as he relaxed into open awareness. His music is described as mathematical intuition and musical inspiration. What wonderful service both these men provided humanity.

A spiritual practice that provides service is called loving kindness meditation or tonglen. This is the simple practice of directing well-wishes towards ourselves and other people. The general idea is to sit comfortably with your eyes closed, and imagine what you wish for your life. Formulate your desires into three or four phrases. Loving-kindness practice is a simple repetition of these phrases, but directing them at different people.

During this practice, become relaxed and open. On the inhale breath, imagine breathing in the suffering and holding the intention that the other (or yourself) is free of suffering. On the exhale breath, offer wellbeing, compassion, peace, harmony and balance for the ones suffering. This intention is put out into the field of consciousness to the intended recipients. I offer a loving kindness practice to those in distress like the people in Haiti following the natural disasters.

Invitation to Practice

To practice loving kindness, sit in a comfortable and relaxed manner. Take two or three deep breaths with slow, long, and complete exhalations. Let go of any concerns or preoccupations. For a few minutes, feel or imagine the breath moving through the center of your chest in the area of your heart. Feel your belly softly rise and fall.

Here is one of many possible loving kindness meditation scripts:

- Take a long and deep breath. As you exhale, smile.
- Scan your body from head to toe and notice any tightness or soreness in any muscle or tissue of the body.
- Breathe into the soreness and soften it. Breathe and let go, so that all the tightness dissolves.

Make these affirmations silently to yourself:

1. May I be safe and protected.
2. May I be happy, peaceful and calm.
3. May I be strong and healthy.
4. May I live with joy and ease.
5. May I be filled with loving kindness.

Visualize a person or people who are suffering. Repeat the affirmations holding the intention of sending loving kindness to them.

1. May they be safe and protected.
2. May they be happy, peaceful and calm.
3. May they be strong and healthy.
4. May they live with joy and ease.
5. May they be filled with loving kindness.

Return to your breath and take a moment to feel gratitude for completing your loving kindness practice.

Amazing research demonstrates our interactions and inter-connections through the field of consciousness, utilizing directed observation and intention. For example, a 1988 study included forty healers directing healing intentions towards forty patients with end stage AIDS. Twenty patients were randomly selected to ten weeks of distant healing treatment and the control group of twenty did not receive distant healing. All other medical care was comparable. The patient population was homogeneous and as similar as statistically possible.

Healers were from Christian, Jewish, Buddhist, Native, American, and shamanic traditions, as well as graduates of secular schools of bioenergetics and meditative healing. Eligibility criteria were a minimum of five years regular ongoing healing practice, previous healing experience at a distance with at least ten patients, and previous healing experience with AIDS. The healers were given a patient's name, photograph, and health details. They were asked to work on the assigned patient for approximately one hour per day for six consecutive days with the instruction to "direct an intention for health and wellbeing" to the subject. The healers treated 5 patients working every other week for 10 weeks of distant healing, each week from a differnt healer. Neither the patients nor the physicians knew which patients received distant healing.

Upon completion of the healing, a blind medical chart review found the patients receiving distant healing acquired significantly fewer new AIDS-defining illnesses, had lower illness severity, required significantly fewer doctor visits and hospitalizations and showed significantly improved mood compared to the control group. In an earlier smaller pilot study four out of ten of the control patients died. In this second longer study 5 percent of the control population died.[6] No deaths occurred in patients receiving distant healing.

This study demonstrates what we know through quantum physics. Energy that exists at the quantum level is not limited in time and space, but exists as a large fluctuating field. When we focus our intention, we shift the energy at the quantum level. A shift at this level affects all other levels in the field. Objects that exist in another level of the field, like molecules and cells, are therefore impacted by our intention. The distant healers were able to focus their intention on an object in the field, the patients, and influence the quantum energy of that object.

We used to believe that we had to be in the same physical location to influence change. In a radical shift of perspective, we are beginning to understand that we can influence that which is non-local (not in our direct individual current time and space) with our intention and attention through the field of consciousness. Our experience of the here and now expands dramatically living in **I am Interconnected**. What we co-create through service at this level of consciousness is no longer limited to our physical location. Service becomes more effective and influential.

In the **I am Infinite** level of consciousness, we live as pure awareness and radiate our presence. We are catalysts for transformation in every moment. Service while living as **I am Infinite**

6. Lynne McTaggart, *The Field: The Quest for the Secret Force of the Universe* (New York: HarperCollins, 2008), 356-63.

ceases being an activity and becomes embedded as a way of living, a natural outpouring of expression with every breath. This is the ultimate service. Service manifests from impulses arising from the fertile ground of all possibility. It may come in any form such as an idea, an opportunity, or an event. If this knowing feels expanding and vitalizing, we give it our attention and intention. This allows the impulse to develop into shape and be expressed in the manifest world. The lived experiences in our lives feels like waves that arise on the sea. Each has a beginning, middle and end. We do not lose the primary identification as the whole sea. We experience the wave, or the manifestation of our individual self, as a temporary form arising from the undifferentiated sea of consciousness.

As I sat in meditation seeking clarity to describe service from **I am Infinite**, the image of a flame appeared. Out of complete nothingness, a flame representing the essence of love arises from the silent intention to be awake. Service occurs out of pure unformed potential of all possibilities. As this flame of love is shared with another, it does not in any way diminish the first flame, but simply spreads light and love. To extend the metaphor, in **I am Interconnected** we see ourselves and others as a candle. At this level, we are also able to serve by finding and sharing the flame of love, but the candle is still our primary identity, separate from others. In **I am Individual** we believe we must give part of our candle and wick to another person in order to share the flame of love with him or her. Thus the flame must be carefully measured and can only be shared with a chosen few.

Our energetic vibration itself positively contributes to the greater good when we embody higher consciousness as it resonates and echoes in the field. Our expanded capacities are expressed directly to the field where other people can "inherit" our wisdom. One term used to describe this phenomenon is morphic resonance, which is the influence of previous structures of activity on subsequent similar structures of activity organized by morphic fields. It enables memories to pass across both space and time from the past. Biological inheritance is not only coded in the genes; much of it depends on morphic resonance from previous members of the species. Thus each individual inherits a collective memory from past members of the species, and also contributes to the collective memory, affecting other members of the species in the future.

A striking experiment involving a long series of tests on rat learning started in Harvard in the 1920s and continued over several decades. Rats learned to escape from a water-maze and subsequent generations learned faster and faster. After the rats learned to escape more than ten times quicker at Harvard, rats tested in Edinburgh, Scotland and in Melbourne, Australia started more or less where the Harvard rats left off. In Melbourne, the rats continued to improve after repeated testing, and this effect was not confined to the descendants of trained rats, suggesting a morphic resonance rather than epigenetic effect.[7]

Spiritual leader Eckhart Tolle invites us to participate in service as **I am Infinite**:

> There is an even deeper level to the whole than interconnectedness of everything in existence. At that deeper level, all

---

7. Rupert Sheldrake, *The Morphic Resonance: The Nature of Formative Causation* (Rochester: Park Street Press, 2009), chapter 11.

things are one. It is the Source, the unmanifested one Life! It is the timeless intelligence that manifests as a universe unfolding in time. The whole is made up of existence and Being, the manifested and unmanifested, the world and God. So when you become aligned with the whole, you become a conscious part of the interconnectedness of the whole and its purpose: the emergence of consciousness into the world.[8]

When my children left home, I made space and time to contemplate the next stage of my life. I reflected on what I wanted to expand in my life and what to let go of that would not serve me going forward. I sold my home and decided to find a place to live that required few resources of time and money. Maybe rent a room from a friend or a small efficiency? It felt like a sabbatical and an adventure. My second intention was to invite more opportunities for teaching, writing, healing, and leading into my life. This made my heart sing just imagining what might arise from the field of infinite possibilities.

It was magical watching the Universe respond. The owner of The Metamorphosis Center, a holistic healing center in my area, called and invited me to present for an evening, which led to offering a four-week class, which led to an all-day conference, which led to monthly teachings, and an invitation to be on the board of directors. When I asked how she found me, she stated my name had come up three different times from people who did not know each other. Each person had recommended me to teach at her center after they had encountered me in various

8. Eckhart Tolle, *A New Earth: Awakening to Your Life's Purpose* (New York: Penguin Books, 2005), 276-277.

areas of my work. She decided to pay attention to the synchronicity and to contact me to participate in her speaker series.

Another service opportunity arose when I was invited to participate in training and creating curriculum for potential new courses offered at the Center for Spirituality & Healing at the University of Minnesota. A brilliant consultant developed an amazing six month training program on Emotional Intelligence and Mindfulness for organizations and leaders. She is retiring soon and shared her wisdom with our small group to utilize in our new program development. There were two other opportunities to teach that developed out this relationship.

I use these skills often in my current coaching practice and have experienced the life-changing shifts people make utilizing these techniques. Mindfulness practices are designed to center, quiet, and open the mind-body-heart and focus attention and awareness in the present moment. These practices also encourage open receptivity, accepting and observing without evaluation or judgment. Through cultivating mindfulness skills, we can decrease stress, gain clarity, enhance creativity and deepen compassion. As we become more mindful, we are more likely to build trust, find common ground, focus on solutions, and make better decisions.

Emotional Intelligence is the ability to know and manage our emotions and be aware of and respond effectively to the emotions of others. As we develop emotional intelligence, we become more self-aware, resilient, socially-aware, empathetic and calm. We improve our capacity to resolve conflict, communicate, engage in meaningful relationships and thrive in change.

Mindfulness and emotional intelligence are a bridge to higher levels of consciousness for those who incorporate these practices in daily living.

These openings came unsolicited and are energizing. They open my imagination and creativity. These circumstances, like all creation, are impermanent, in flux, and transient. The underlying energy that created them remains constant. Yes, I have connected with amazing like-hearted and like-minded people through my involvement in these projects, which I savor. Yet, I know these opportunities will also have a beginning, middle, and end. I am not attaching my identity to belonging to the particular programs or organizations. This gives me freedom to immerse myself fully into the moments when I am developing a class or workshop, writing or teaching. I allow the Divine spark that lives in my **Center Within** to express itself fully in these activities without attachment to their longevity or recognition. My presence rests in the unchanging state of being that all form and events arise from.

I had several other invitations to work on potentially impactful service projects. They felt exciting, and my ego was very impressed by one in particular. After resting in quiet reflection, considering each one as they were presented, I turned down the others. They were not fully aligned with what makes my heart sing. What I say "No" to is just as important as what I say "Yes" to. I invite you to be open to the miracles of opportunity for service that arise in your life, and say yes to those which align with your heart.

Gift of Transformation

We are living amidst a transformative period in human development, experiencing dramatic paradigm shifts, exponential acceleration, and leaps in human consciousness itself. It is exhilarating and it is terrifying. Humanity is at a crossroads. We must choose to cease our *doing* that fosters depletion, conflict, separation, and scarcity, and choose to support *being* sustainable, collaborative, inclusive, and abundant. When in fear, we allow limiting ideas, beliefs, self-talk and disease generated from ourselves or others to direct our experience. When living from our gifts, talents, passions, and strengths, we consciously co-create who we are becoming personally, interpersonally, professionally and collectively. Living in our power as the full expression of our true nature from our **Center Within** is a treasured gift to all beings.

Reflection

Describe a time you were involved in service as **I am Individual**. Were there any strings attached, a sense of debt owed from the giver to the receiver, or an entitled right for the giver to impose their views on the receiver?

Remember a time when you have received service from the perspective of **I am Interconnected**. How did you experience the contribution from this person's passion, essence, and authenticity?

What activities of service in your life give you energy and feel expansive?

When have you chosen to say no to an invitation to participate in a worthy activity because it felt constricting or not in alignment with your authentic self?

PART TWO

THE TRUTH: BECOMING WHOLE

CHAPTER SIX

INCREASING SELF-AWARENESS

Using a witness perspective to build self-awareness is essential in moving towards higher consciousness where I see you seeing me, knowing we, and being Thee.

The first step towards living in higher consciousness is assessing our condition. We have explored the condition of human beings and various structures in our world. We have discussed strategies for examining our inner and outer selves. There is transformation occurring in and around us, and we can co-create a world that supports the highest good for all beings. We can make choices that encourage transparency, compassion, interdependence, abundance and sustainability. Through the wisdom of ancient teachings and modern insights we can make the shift to collective higher consciousness. As always, this process begins with each of us. As Mahatma Gandhi told us:

> We but mirror the world. All the tendencies present in the outer world are to be found in the world of our body. If we could change ourselves, the tendencies in the world would

also change. As a man changes his own nature, so does the attitude of the world change towards him. This is the divine mystery supreme. A wonderful thing it is and the source of our happiness. We need not wait to see what others do.[9]

One way to change ourselves is increasing our ability to assess our condition. We can do this by being more self-aware. Increasing our self-awareness is essential in moving to higher levels of consciousness. Once we notice our own reactivity, thoughts, body sensations, and emotions we can utilize practices such as loving kindness to enhance our ability to remain calm and choose our response in any experience. The first step is realizing our condition in the present moment.

Take a few minutes to notice your body, thoughts, and emotions. Take a deep breath and bring all of your attention into your body. Scan your body slowly from head to toe with attention. Where is your body tight, in pain, or feeling constricted? How relaxed are your shoulders, tongue, lower back, hips and ankles? Calm and soften your body as deeply as you can.

Next, notice what you are thinking about. Take a deep breath and bring all of your attention to your thoughts. Are your thoughts in the present moment or are they off on a tangent thinking about something that is not actually occurring now? Are your thoughts focused on the past or what ifs in the future? When your thoughts are engaged in worry or rumination, your attention is not available for the present moment.

Assess your emotional condition. Take a deep breath and

9. Mahatma Gandhi, *The Collected Works of M. K. Gandhi* (New Delhi: The Publications Division, 1913), 241.

bring all of your attention to your emotions. What do you feel? Are you anxious, optimistic, calm, irritable, alert, curious, angry, happy, or sad? Does your emotional state have anything to do with what is happening in the present moment? If you find you're emotionally reactive to something that is not presently occurring, refocus your attention to the here and now.

Invitation to Practice

Take 60 seconds three times a day to relax and put your attention on your present condition. Find one minute in the morning, one minute during the day and one minute before bed to scan your body, thoughts, and emotions.

- Begin by taking a few deep clearing breaths. Bring all of our attention into the present moment.

- What do you notice?

- Scan your body. Are there spots that are tight? Soften and relax them with your attention and intention.

- Scan your thoughts. Lean into the viewpoint that is observing the thoughts and not caught in them. Can you shift your perspective to this neutral watcher anytime you choose?

- Scan your emotions. What words describe your feelings? Are they attached to a past or possible future experience?

Return your attention to your breathing and relax your entire body.

We can only make the choice to relax more fully if we are first self-aware of any unhealthy or unnecessary constriction in our physical, mental, and emotional body.

One technique we can utilize to bring our attention more fully into this moment is assessing our five senses. What are you hearing, seeing, smelling, touching, and tasting? Allow your awareness to be open and alert in this moment. Maintaining optimal balance in mind, body, and emotions frees up attention and expands our awareness.

Another way to increase our self-awareness is observing stress in our lives. What symptoms do you notice in your body when you are stressed? Tight shoulders, stomach ache, grinding teeth? How does your behavior change when you are stressed? Biting nails, retreating, change in sleep patterns, eating more or less, crying easily, medicating, or distracting yourself? How do you emotionally react when you are stressed? Are you quick to become angry, annoyed, numb or withdrawn? Do you feel more suspicious, jealous, shut down, anxious or depressed?

If we live in a continuous state of high arousal we will develop chronic symptoms of an overactive stress response. The stress response is a natural reaction in our body's nervous and chemical systems designed to protect us from harm. Our respiratory rate increases, blood is directed to our muscles and limbs, pupils dilate, pulse quickens, and our focus and awareness intensifies as we prepare for fight or flight. Left unchecked, this leads to exaggerated fear, distorted thinking, hyper-vigilance, burnout, and dis-ease.

Another technique for developing self-awareness is

identifying stressful triggers. Internal activities such as worrying about the past or future, negative self-talk, or limiting beliefs can trigger the stress response. It becomes activated even if we are only imagining a triggering event! When we catch ourselves worrying about a stressor that is not actually occurring in the present moment, we can change that thought and the resulting emotional response. The stress response stops when we remove our attention from a worrisome thought, which allows our mind-body to return to balance.

External circumstances can be stressors also. If we become aware of our body, thoughts, or emotions reacting with hyper-arousal automatically to an outside irritation, we can learn to relax and constructively engage rather than being dictated by a conditioned stress reaction. Self-awareness of internal and external stressors empowers us to choose our response. We can avoid and prevent stress triggers when possible, and cope more effectively when they occur.

This is easier said than done. When my son was in grade school, we stopped one Saturday at the bank to pick up a cashier's check I needed later that day to buy a used car from a private seller. We were running on a tight schedule. I was completely frustrated when the bank teller said the funds I had transferred into my account a few days earlier were not available yet. I requested she find a way to make them accessible immediately. As she went to find her supervisor, I walked over to get a cup of water and attempted to calm down. When I returned to her teller window, she repeated that I did not have enough funds available for the cashier check. I was engulfed in rage. As I continued my protest, I set the cup of water down with so much force the water flew out of the cup and all over the teller. I did not notice my pulse racing, my teeth clenching, my hands sweating nor my son slithering towards to door utterly embarrassed. What if I could have noticed my stress response escalating towards that moment? Could I have made a choice to respond differently rather than be overwhelmed with reactivity?

An important key to self-awareness is the capacity to clearly assess our condition in the present moment. This requires developing an observer, witness, or watcher perspective. From an observer perspective, we "see" ourselves in a reaction. We simply notice it without judgment. This allows us to observe ourselves honestly. It is important to learn which things we have the ability to control, and which we do not, and not to become angry at others when things do not immediately go our way. The capacity to observe what is actually occurring without imposing false beliefs, judgment, or negative self-talk is a treasured gift to yourself (and your family, friends, and colleagues!) in the process of waking up into higher consciousness.

A Taoist teaching about a Chinese farmer illustrates the observer concept. He attached no reaction or distorted meaning to what was occurring in his life:

> This farmer had only one horse, and one day the horse ran away. The neighbors came to console him over his terrible loss. The farmer said, "What makes you think it is so terrible?" A month later, the horse came home, this time bringing with her two beautiful wild horses. The neighbors became excited at the farmer's good fortune. Such lovely strong horses! The farmer said, "What makes you think

this is good fortune?" The farmer's son was thrown from one of the wild horses and broke his leg. All the neighbors were very distressed. Such bad luck! The farmer said, "What makes you think it is bad?" A war came, and every able-bodied man was conscripted and sent into battle. Only the farmer's son, because he had a broken leg, remained. The neighbors congratulated the farmer. "What makes you think this is good?" said the farmer.[10]

Invitation to Practice

- Set time aside for alert, open, nonjudgmental self-reflection to observe thoughts, emotions, and behaviors you had throughout the day in order to gain deeper insight to stress symptoms and triggers.

- Make a list of the physical, emotional, mental and behavioral responses you have when you get stressed. See if you can notice them throughout the day as soon as they begin. Practice relaxing and refocusing your attention into the present moment.

- Make a list of your stress triggers. What internal activities and external circumstances turn your stress response on? Which ones can you prevent or avoid? Practice relaxing and refocusing your attention into the present moment.

How would our capacity to stay calm, open, and present be affected if we could observe our life with the Chinese farmer's

---

10. Elise Hancock, "Editor's Note," *Johns Hopkins Magazine*, November (1993), 2.

clarity? When we develop a witness or observer perspective, we can notice ourselves in a reaction. The witness is like a mirror. It is a neutral observer watching our reactions as if it were looking at an object. Not good or bad, just what is. In the beginning, we may only be able to observe a reaction after the stress response has subsided. As this skill develops, we learn to observe the physical, emotional, and mental stress symptoms as they begin. This gives us the option to relax, avoid, or reverse our reactivity and choose an appropriate response.

Another way to visualize the experience of shifting between having a reaction and observing our reaction is to imagine viewing a magic eye picture. Have you ever looked at a magic eye picture? At first the image appears to be a design of squiggly lines of various colors. When you shift your focus with your eyes, a three dimensional picture comes into view. If you can keep this soft focus, the picture remains. If you return your eyes to a hard focus, you lose the three dimensional picture. When you are living in **I am Individual,** using the witness or observer perspective allows you to cultivate the soft focus or subject perspective so you can see additional layers and dimensions.

Our witness or observer self develops with practice. We will notice with more frequency physical sensations, memories, emotions, thoughts, energetic experience, and intuition in the moment as they are occurring. We gain the ability to have two simultaneous perspectives of having a reaction and observing the reaction without judgment. We have a sense of powerlessness if we live with an underlying fear that, at any moment, an internal thought or belief or an external stimulus can trigger a reaction that makes us feel out of control. We feel like a victim at the mercy of our own reactivity.

However, as our witness or observer is cultivated, we recognize these triggers and reactions in the moment more easily as they arise. Then we have a choice and can take responsibility for the consequences of our perceptions. We can choose how to respond rather than get caught up in the reaction. We have the ability and freedom to choose to respond from the witness perspective confidently rather than feel like a victim and have our behavior dictated by reactivity. Our witness or observer provides insight into understanding our tendencies, resistances, preferences, idealizations, beliefs, and patterns.

Some years ago I managed four branches of a nationwide company that served twelve Midwestern states and provided intravenous medication to patients in their homes. We were having a national meeting to discuss a plan to move our billing departments from local service areas to one centralized site. As the morning progressed, it became apparent the corporate department making the strategic plan to consolidate our billing processes did not understand the nuances and vast differences between local insurance company requirements. As I got more agitated, I asked several challenging questions that exposed the lack of knowledge of the team presenting.

During our lunch break, I was venting to one of my colleagues. She was an excellent listener and validated my frustration. She was compassionate and she was able to feel and understand me without needing to fix, judge, or change me or the situation. Being with me and my hostility, she offered a suggestion I have never forgotten. My morning contributions to the meeting may have been right, but they were not kind. She challenged me to be right and kind. This would require more self-awareness, staying calm and quiet inside, observing and witnessing without evaluation or judgment. Could I choose to respond with kindness instead of react out of my annoyance?

The afternoon went much better. When I noticed my stress response rise, I was able to take a few deep breaths and bring my attention back into the present moment. Only when I was calm did I choose to patiently offer questions and suggestions that would benefit all involved in the process. We built trust and respect for each other's ideas and different opinions. In the end the company made the "right" choice and never did centralize billing. It felt great to harness my passion and expertise productively instead of arrogantly and sarcastically.

As the holes and wounds that get triggered begin to heal through our deepening insights, we begin to notice even more clearly that there are patterns and connections in our reactions. As our witness reflects like a mirror, observing without judgment, being compassionate, we can relate a reaction in this moment to similar circumstances and experience in our past. Recognizing parallel responses to internal or external triggers over time can provide insight into underlying beliefs, holes, and embellished meaning. This self-awareness allows us to heal, grow, release, and neutralize reactivity. We move closer to being whole.

Once we can live reliably in our centered mind-body with reliable access to our witness perspective, we can explore more expansive levels of self. Wholeness is a quality of a person whose identity resides in **I am Interconnected**. If we live at this level of consciousness, we can sustain open access to our witness observer. Judgment falls away and is replaced by discernment. We observe the present moment without adding inaccurate meaning. We can see all sides of an issue clearly.

The sense of separation and duality appearing right or wrong, good or bad, softens into understanding differentiation and variety on a continuum. We spend less time with our stress response turned on and more time relaxing. At this level our witness perspective observes as we increase our free attention and open awareness.

Continuing this practice of observing and reflecting, we ultimately open to realize that which contains both the object and subject. Duality disappears and we experience the energy of pure awareness from which all arises. This is sometimes referred to as the Void, Ground of Being, All That Is, or Unknowable Potential. Resting here, **I am Infinite** is experienced. The perspective beyond the mirror itself is the essence of all the seen and unseen world. We know all levels of consciousness simultaneously. I see you seeing me, knowing we, and being Thee. We are pure essence expressing as each miraculous iteration of form in the vast sea of consciousness.

Reflection

Recall a time you over-reacted. What was the trigger? What did you notice in your body, thoughts, and emotions? How did you bring yourself back to balance?

What steps can you take to develop your witness observer, that part of you watching without judgment when you have physical and emotional reactions?

What is your experience when your individual body, mind, or emotions are in balance and require little attention?

There are many techniques that we can use to become calm and at peace. What are your favorite ways to quiet your body, mind, and emotions to experience deep stillness?

Can you identify your false beliefs, self-judgment, or negative self-talk that lead to assumptions like the Chinese farmer's neighbor?

CHAPTER SEVEN

TRANSFORMING PRACTICES

Transforming practices assist us individually and collectively in moving from dysfunctional to functional, from functional to optimal, and from optimal to enlightened.

Human beings are miraculously engineered. With our attention and intention, we are able to activate the relaxation response, a state of deep rest that changes the physical and emotional fight or flight responses to stress. When we relax, we counteract the hypervigilant responses of stress by decreasing blood pressure, respiratory rate, and pulse rate. In addition, we slow down the aging process, reduce anxiety, improve sleep, increase emotional calm and reverse distorted thinking and fear.

Relaxing influences important change at the cellular level in our bodies. In every human cell we find mitochondria. They convert chemical energy from food into a form that cells can use. They also maintain control of cell health and growth. Activating the relaxation response improves mitochondrial energy production and utilization and promotes mitochondrial resiliency.

Relaxing also improves our insulin secretion and reduces the expression of genes in our cells linked to inflammatory response and stress related pathways.

Epigenetics is the study of changes in gene expression (active or expressing versus inactive or not expressing genes) without the underlying DNA sequence changing. Epigenetic change is a regular and natural occurrence, but can also be influenced by factors including stress, age, the environment, lifestyle, and disease state. Biological inheritance is not only coded in the genes, or in epigenetic modifications of the genes; much of it depends on morphic resonance from previous members of the species.

Telomeres protect the end of the chromosome from deterioration in a manner similar to the way the tips of shoelaces keep them from unraveling. When we produce relaxation hormones and chemicals, the telomeres are better maintained, improving long-term cell health. Our cells also become more efficient in their oxygen consumption and carbon dioxide elimination.

Activating the relaxation response increases the growth of high functioning brain cells and connections. When people do relaxation exercises, growth has been measured in the cortex region which is located in the front and outer parts of the brain. Growth in both the number of brain cells and the number of connections between brain cells has been observed. This part of the brain is associated with memory, attention, perception, awareness, thought, and language. Monitoring advanced meditators' brains while they are meditating shows increased cortex brain activity over a control group of people who do not meditate. Activating the relaxation response literally transforms us at a cellular level to become higher functioning!

So what are these relaxation-eliciting practices? Transforming practices are activities designed to center, quiet, and open the mind-body-heart. They help us focus attention and awareness in the present moment. These mindfulness practices encourage open receptivity, accepting and observing without evaluation or judgment.

Transforming practices accelerate the natural unfolding process of human development. Our awareness expands, revealing our true nature in higher consciousness. Depending on our present condition, transforming practices can have many purposes. According to fabulous research on transformation presented by Marilyn Schlitz et al. (2007):

> Transforming practices quiet the mind-body, heal old wounds, shed false beliefs, cultivate intention and attention, promote insight, and expand capacities. The heart of these practices is their ability to bring you into direct contact with the numinous, open your eyes and heart to the sanctity of life. They assist you in realizing the abundant, ever-present, and surprisingly accessible deep meaning that is present in every moment of every day.[11]

What are examples of these transforming practices? They include but are not limited to:

---

11. Marilyn Schlitz, *Living Deeply: The Art and Science of Transformation in Everyday Life* (Oakland: New Harbinger Publications, 2007), 104.

- Breath work: patterns of breathing
- Meditation: mindfulness, concentrative, moving, open
- Music: listening to chant, singing, toning
- Silence: being in quiet
- Smell: aromatherapy
- Mindful eating: intentionally prepare and eat a meal
- Vision: screen savers, wall colors, art, photographs, decorating your spaces, creating vision boards
- Feng Shui: creating harmonious environments
- Body Movement: exercise, yoga, qi gong, tai chi, stretch, walk a labyrinth, dance
- Guided Imagery: autogenics, visualizations
- Journal: writing and reflecting, creating a gratitude journal
- Art: writing, drawing, sculpting, creating mandalas, making collages
- Biofeedback: using instruments that provide feedback on physiological changes
- Progressive relaxation: contracting and relaxing muscles sequentially from head to toes
- Being in nature: walking, sitting, observing
- Reflection: contemplating and studying: sacred text, poetry, koans, myths, symbols, metaphor, archetypes

- Ritual: sequence of activities involving gestures, words, and objects that support an intention
- Dialogue: speaking and listening authentically and deeply
- Dreams: recording, contemplating, exploring meaning and insights in dreams
- Storytelling: examining current story, creating new story

Transforming practices can be utilized in our day-to-day activities. For instance, during a morning shower, practice focusing your attention using all five senses to feel the warm water on the skin, smell the soap, hear the soothing water, see the colors and light, and maybe taste a bit of the fresh water. Notice how paying attention with all five senses brings your attention into the present moment.

We have examined incorporating reflecting on your present condition throughout the day using our witness perspective. We can bring our observer viewpoint to every moment and notice what is occurring in our body, mind and heart. If we notice a stress symptom, we can do a quick practice such as stretching or walking in nature. This will bring our attention into the present moment and activate the relaxation response.

I had a client who utilized his witness perspective to observe his stress response and triggers each day. Upon reflection, he realized he became stressed several times a day at work. This diminished his productivity and creativity. To reverse his stress response, he took deep long breaths for sixty seconds. He changed his screen saver to a picture from his favorite vacation spot and added an inspiring quote. When possible, he mindfully packs his lunch and eats outside alone. Transforming practice can reverse the stress response and quickly returns our mind-body to balance.

Ritual is a powerful transforming practice. We incorporate ritual into our celebrations, holidays, worship, and rites of passage. They can be included in our daily routine also. We can create a small space in our home or office that holds a photograph or object that reminds us of an intention we set. I remember a vacation with dear friends and family in Seattle where we spent a day on Vashon Island. We walked Point Robinson Park, and I had a conversation with one of my friends. She suddenly had an epiphany, a deep intuitive insight into the topic we were discussing.

Strolling down the beach alone contemplating this new understanding, she spontaneously added a ritual by picking up a small rock as a keepsake. It reminds her of the revelation and her intention to integrate this new awareness into her daily living.

The next day we went to the farmers market and she was telling me about the rock she was carrying in her pocket. She stated an intention to have it made into a necklace to honor the moment and further remind her of the gem of wisdom she had discovered. We had stopped in front of a booth where a woman was wrapping stones and making pendants. Ten minutes later she was wearing her rock, now a piece of jewelry, around her neck. Adding a ritual, gesture, word, or object that supports our intention can enhance our experience. Ritual can assist us in remaining open to a new, larger worldview and in having greater access to the field of consciousness.

Bedtime is another wonderful time to add a transforming practice to your daily routine. We can take a few moments to reflect on our day and recall three times we were grateful. Scientific studies on people who intentionally cultivate thankfulness have proven these people experience more positive emotions, feel more alive, sleep better, express more compassion and kindness, and have stronger immune systems. Deep sleep is essential to restore our minds and bodies to balance every night. Practices such as progressive relaxation and listening to calming music can improve our sleep. Guided imagery, proactively focusing and directing your imagination in positive ways, can also be a powerful bedtime practice. You can image yourself at your favorite vacation spot or imagine your muscles softening and relaxing. There are many recorded guided imageries with words and music available. You will find resources such as guided imagery on my website.

Keep the practices embedded in your routine simple. Invite them to enhance your day, not be a stressor or a burden. Practice in various ways and follow what calls to you. Change them up and be playful and curious. Make them part of your everyday life. Our breath is free and always available to elicit the relaxation response. You can take a few deep breaths or practice various rhythmic breathing patterns for calming and creating openings to higher levels of consciousness.

It is also valuable to set aside practice time from our daily routine to relax and reflect. We can take a walk in nature or partake in a yoga, exercise, qi gong, tai chi, or dance class. We can record our dreams and spend time reading and reflecting on them to see if they reveal an insight or revelation. Reading sacred texts has been important in every wisdom tradition. Hinduism, Buddhism, Christianity, Judaism, Taoism, Confucianism, and Islam are just some of the religions that have beautiful teachings on higher levels of consciousness worthy of contemplation. Poetry can also inspire us to deeper levels. Transforming practices support us at every stage of development: healing holes when we live at **I am Individual**, becoming whole at **I am Interconnected** and being Holy at **I am Infinite**.

Retreats encourage mindful activities set aside from our daily routine. I facilitate workshops that give participants an opportunity to immerse in transforming practices for a day or two. At a recent workshop, we spent an afternoon creating collages from magazine images and words on index cards. We used a number of transforming practices woven into our day. At the beginning of our collage process, we did a body scan to notice tight areas in our bodies and then imagined them soften and relax. We energized our bodies, minds, hearts and space with gratitude. During the afternoon we alternated between silence and healing music. We utilized essential oils in a diffuser to aid our relaxation.

We spent some time reflecting on our collages when they were complete. One of the women noticed a pattern in her collage. Words and images about fun and riches were often hidden by restricting images like boulders, bars or fences. Through storytelling, she uncovered a belief that she does not feel worthy of abundance. With that powerful untrue story revealed, she was able to re-enter her life paying attention to opportunities for joy, wealth and ease while eliminating self-sabotaging behaviors that kept her in lack or scarcity. As I stayed in touch with her through individual coaching sessions, I was delighted to see her make small changes in her lifestyle which improved her health and wellbeing. She began to say yes to opportunities and relationships that expanded her work. Her business thrived and prospered.

There are some transforming practices thought to be more body-centered, mind-centered, or heart-centered. All practices impact all of these aspects of our human being, but some put more emphasis on one aspect. We can choose a practice that focuses on the body, mind or heart.

If you are a body way person, someone who enjoys getting into the flow or the zone through exercise or dance, for instance, you may find mindful movement, progressive relaxation or being in nature the easiest way to practice. Scanning your entire body slowly from the tips of your toes to the top of your head, feeling every somatic sensation can bring you fully into the present moment. Resting your attention on each area, imagining them soften and relax and breathing deeply may effortlessly quiet your thoughts, feelings, and physical body.

If you are a heart way person, feeling the flow when you are in service to others may open you to new levels of awareness. If you are feeling moved by the suffering of others you may find chant, loving kindness practice, or storytelling beneficial. Cultivating gratitude in your life can enhance your wellbeing.

Practicing compassion can be inviting and natural to a heart way person.

If you are a mind way person, someone who enjoys learning new ways or intellectual discussions, you may find that contemplating and studying sacred text, poetry, koans, myths, symbols, metaphor, or archetypes expand your awareness and activate the relaxation response. You may find paying attention to your dreams enlightening. The witness observer can be useful as you notice your reactivity or desire to avoid or attach, which takes your mind out of the present moment.

Invitation to practice

- Choose one transforming practice you will use throughout your day if you notice your stress response turning on.

- Choose one transforming practice you will use for 60 seconds a day when you are free from reactivity to deepen your relaxation response.

- Once a week, set aside 30 minutes to engage in a transforming practice.

Strengthen your skills of transforming practices by regularly utilizing the ones that feel the most inviting. In addition, try new techniques. Add them to your daily routine and set aside time to immerse yourself in relaxation. Over time, as your baseline state of consciousness expands, your practices will shift and change also. Allow the best practice for you to arise from your wisdom by routinely assessing of your present condition.

Reflection

Describe an experience you had using a relaxation practice in the moment when you were stressed or reactive. Did it bring you back to balance?

What are your favorite transforming practices to relax and to open you to new insights and expand your perspective?

When did you experience a transforming practice open you up to a new insight or expand your perspective?

Have you heard about a new practice you would like to learn more about and to try?

Have you been on a retreat or workshop that was impactful in your life? Do you have any scheduled in the near future?

How can you learn about organizations or people in your area who will support you in learning new practices?

CHAPTER EIGHT

SUPPORTING THE JOURNEY

Coaches assist us in assimilating, integrating, and stabilizing higher consciousness and can be invaluable on the journey.

We live in a time when we have access to many resources. Through the Internet, we can read emerging knowledge, take classes from teachers all over the world, or research any topic we choose. Yet information alone is insufficient for integrating and embodying wisdom into our daily lives. Connecting with other people who are living at higher level of consciousness is essential for lasting transformation.

It can be useful to share our experiences with a supportive community of like-minded and like-hearted people. We can find companions for the journey in formal religious settings like churches, mosques, temples, or synagogues. There are local and national organizations that meet online, in small groups, and at national conferences communicating and learning about various types of transforming practices. There are classes and workshops available through academic institutions and independent teachers, healers, and leaders. There are websites, books, podcasts, webinars, and DVDs. There are social media groups.

It can be easier to maintain unity awareness in groups where everyone is actively choosing to be self-aware and discovering their highest levels of consciousness. When I teach transforming practices, for example, it is easier for me to feel no separation of myself as teacher, the students, and the teachings that are being practiced. Out of nothing comes the flow of our activities, moment to moment. As I explore higher consciousness with like-minded people, new frontiers of subtle energy, vibration, and knowing are revealed. The community supports my awakening more fully. It deepens my experience of my essence of pure spirit which manifests as me, we, and Thee expressing in the world.

There are also many mind-body-spirit practitioners who offer supportive services. They include, but are not limited to, massage therapists, nutritionists, energy healers, mental health providers, primary care providers, chiropractors, spiritual directors, acupuncturists, aromatherapists, traditional Chinese medicine providers, and homoeopaths. By trusting ourselves in the process, we will discover communities and teachers who can serve us perfectly as we unfold into deeper realization.

Coaches offer companionship and guidance along the journey. A transformational coach assists clients in realizing and developing self-directed plans to explore avenues of growth and to implement the changes they desire. Coaches are trained in various aspects and levels of consciousness, human development, transforming practices, and coaching techniques. During coaching sessions, the locus of expertise lies in the client and the process is collaborative and co-creative. All good coaches practice and integrate these skills and ways of knowing into their own daily living.

Coaches create conditions that increase the likelihood that transformation will occur as new levels of awareness and consciousness reveal themselves to a client. This is done by creating sacred space and a protective container through such activities such as deep listening, reframing, encouraging, witnessing, and maintaining confidentiality. The coach and client develop a sacred trust through transparency and vulnerability. They work together to uncover, identify, and heal the client's holes and move towards becoming whole. A coach can support a client's processes until they are aware of themselves as **I am Interconnected** and **I am Infinite**. The self-directed plans and steps the coach and client co-create are a personalized map to living in a state of higher consciousness.

Also, a coach can see his or her client's potential fully realized even if the client cannot yet see it for him or herself. Similar to our inner witness observing our thoughts, feelings, beliefs, and self-talk, a coach can also offer this feedback from an observer perspective. A coach can reframe a client's way of viewing and experiencing events, ideas, concepts, and emotions to find more positive alternatives. This can expedite a client's ability to see his or her circumstance from another perspective. This poem simply and eloquently illustrates how our experiences and choices are dramatically impacted by our outlook and evaluation of our circumstances.

An Autobiography in 5 Short Chapters

Chapter One
I walk down the street.
There is a deep hole in the sidewalk.
I fall in.
I am lost...I am helpless.
It isn't my fault.
It takes forever to find a way out.

Chapter Two
I walk down the same street.
There is a deep hole in the sidewalk.
I pretend I don't see it.
I fall in again.
I can't believe I am in the same place,
But it isn't my fault.
It still takes a long time to get out.

Chapter Three
I walk down the same street.
There is a deep hole in the sidewalk.
I see it there.
I still fall in...it's a habit.
But my eyes are open.
I know where I am.
It is my fault.
I get out immediately.

Chapter Four
I walk down the same street.
There is a deep hole in the sidewalk.
I walk around it.

Chapter Five
I walk down another street.[12]

We can walk down the same street falling in the same rut or hole without recognizing the many choices we have available to us. Coaches can challenge limiting beliefs and negative self-talk such as, "I am helpless" or "It is not my fault." We often fall into habits and assess new situations based on our previous experience. The feelings, thoughts, sensations, and muscle actions of every event become embedded in our network of brain cells. Every time we repeat a particular thought or action, we strengthen the connection between a set of brain cells. The neurons that fire together get wired together. The brain continuously lays down neurological tracks that link particular emotions and body sensations with particular situations. We can find ourselves in a personally created loop.

This firing together is what makes habits difficult to break. We need to separate out the various wires the way an electrician might, by pulling them apart and permanently tying them off. This disconnects the habits we don't want to keep. We replace the old linkage with new associations that enforce more functional

---

12. Portia Nelson, *There's a Hole in My Sidewalk: The Romance of Self-Discovery* (Hillsboro: Beyond Words Publishing Inc), 2-3. Used with permission.

and optimal habits. We rewire our brains and bodies and lay down new tracks that support our opening to higher levels of consciousness. Coaches can help us see and break free from our conditioning and habits.

Habits are another reason transforming practices are so important. Raising awareness of what we are doing while we are doing it will help us to make thoughtful choices impacting us behaviorally, cognitively and somatically. We create new habits by expanding our awareness and accessing higher levels of consciousness.

In addition to recognizing habits, a coach can also assist a client in identifying his or her present level of consciousness. The transforming practices we choose at each level of consciousness are designed to promote fulfillment at the current level and open awareness to include the next level. Living as **I am Individual,** we often identify holes appearing as wounds, distortions, guilt, confusion, shame, or stagnation. If we utilize practices designed to address our wounds, we often reduce stress, improve physical health, and enhance relaxation. If our minds are obsessing over an event in the past or future, a coach may recommend a concentrative practice to remove our attention from rumination and worry and redirect it into the present moment.

Learning to self-regulate is a goal of this level of consciousness. Self-regulation is the ability to monitor and control our own behavior, emotions, or thoughts. It is the ability to calm ourselves down when we are upset and cheer ourselves up when we are down. Self-regulation is also the ability to act in our long-term best interest, consistent with our deepest values.

For this level of consciousness, as a coach I may recommend a practice to focus our attention and relax such as:

- Walking and moving mindfully
- Focusing on the breath
- Listening to a guided imagery meditation
- Listening to balancing music
- Smelling aromatherapy
- Progressive relaxation
- Being in nature

All of these practices increase our capacity to self-regulate in the moment and move towards wholeness.

Invitation to Practice

Autogenic Biofeedback

- Scan your body and choose 5 parts of your body that feel tight or sore. Choose one of your identified areas and imagine it relaxing and softening.

- Choose a phrase that names the body part and follow it by two words such as soft, heavy, warm, relaxed, or still. Slowly and silently repeat each phrase 4 times, pausing a few seconds between each repetition.

- Use guided imagery to image your chosen body part becoming soft, heavy, warm, relaxed, still, or whatever words you chose to use in your phrase.

- Focus on a second area of the body and repeat this process with a new phrase.

- Repeat with each body area.

- When complete, take a deep breath in and out and smile.

Examples include:

- My feet feel heavy and still.

- My belly and lower back feel warm and soft.

- My arms and shoulders feel limp and relaxed.

- My neck and jaw feel open and calm.

Once we have stability living in our centered body-mind, we can change the focus of our practice towards self-exploration and being part of the whole. We explore vastness and the yet unrealized potential in ourselves through unfocused and non-judgmental mediation. This can provide a clearer lens in which to experience new levels of ourselves. When we contemplate and reflect, we expand our awareness to connections and patterns in ourselves and throughout the sea of consciousness. Practices that open our awareness rather than focus our concentration can be more useful here.

As a coach, I may recommend transforming practices such as:

- Journaling

- Creating collage

- Chanting

- Studying symbol, myth, dreams, poetry, sacred texts, metaphor, archetype

- Practicing ritual

When clients live primarily in **I am Interconnected** identity, we work together to develop personal insight, present-moment awareness, open-hearted wakefulness and self-understanding. As self-awareness can be developed as illustrated in *An Autobiography in 5 Short Chapters,* we can also notice each other's holes and assist by pointing them out or filling them in for each other. All of these practices lead to increasing sensitivity to subtle energy and patterns that have always existed, but were outside their perception. Revelation, synchronicity, and intuition become more accessible. Clients explore many ways of knowing themselves at new levels of awareness.

Another tool for self-exploration is contemplating and practicing inner qualities and attitudes. Many timeless wisdom traditions encourage developing these higher consciousness abilities also. The Christian tradition offers the seven virtues of prudence, justice, temperance (or restraint), courage, faith, hope, and charity (or love). Buddhism offers the Noble Eightfold Path and Four Noble Truths. Other qualities worth cultivating include tolerance, forgiveness, hope, altruism, forgiveness, compassion, honesty, creativity, balance, resilience, patience, acceptance, openness, empathy, love, kindness, acceptance, forgiveness, appreciation, equanimity, and open-heartedness.

When a client has access to **I am Infinite**, he or she moves towards the goal of self-liberation, transcending or dis-identifying from the sense of being a separate self. He or she develop a sense of harmony with the universe. Cultivating practice with this focus increases our compassion, sensitivity, and service towards others. Transforming practices may include any or all of the activities as each higher level of consciousness always include all previous realized levels.

Invitation to Practice

Choose one of the following qualities and focus on practicing it continuously for two days. Write and/or draw about your experience. You can repeat this exercise, changing words every two days. Add qualities you would like to expand in your own life.

Qualities of **I am Interconnected:**

- Non-judging: impartial witnessing, observing the present, moment by moment without evaluation and categorization

- Non-striving: non-goal oriented, remaining unattached to outcome or achievement, not forcing things

- Acceptance: open to seeing and acknowledging things as they are in the present moment. Acceptance does not mean passivity or resignation, rather a clearer understanding of the present so one can more effectively respond

- Patience: allowing things to unfold in their time, bringing patience to ourselves, to others, and to the present moment

- Trust: trusting both oneself, one's body, intuition, emotions, as well as trusting that life is unfolding as it is supposed to

- Openness: seeing things as if for the first time, creating possibility by paying attention to all feedback in the present moment

- Letting go: non-attachment, not holding on to thoughts, feelings, experiences; this does not mean suppressing

- Gentleness: characterized by a soft, considerate and tender quality; this is not passive, undisciplined or indulgent

- Generosity: giving in the present moment within a context of love and compassion, without attachment to gain or thought of return

- Compassion: the quality of feeling and understanding another person's situation in the present moment, his or her perspectives, emotions, actions, and being with them without needing to fix, judge, or change the person or the situation

- Gratitude: the quality of reverence, appreciating and being thankful for the present moment

- Loving kindness: a quality embodying benevolence, compassion and cherishing; a quality filled with forgiveness and unconditional love

Eventually, transforming practices cease being activities and become embedded as a way of living moment to moment, a natural outpouring of expression with every breath. This radical shift from doing to being leads to the fulfillment of this level of consciousness, a sense of oneness in our unique expression, complete liberation. There is lived experience of the self as Holy. This level of awareness is still uncommon among people and often appears outside of acceptable norms and values of society. Working with a coach can validate and ease this transition as clients embody **I am Infinite** identity.

Coaches assist clients to understand, integrate and embody new experiences and realizations. They can examine current and falling-away paradigms together. Occasionally, transforming experiences can be unsettling. They can feel out of the ordinary as we move into unknown territory. Gradual emergence of new paradigms and perspectives is preferred to becoming overwhelmed, which can cause disruption in our psychological, social, and occupational functioning. It is important for clients to stay centered amidst openings to new views of reality that often do not fit with the dominant cultural model of what is true and acceptable.

I had a client who explained to me the colors and patterns he sees around people. It was so outside of his beliefs about reality that he had never spoken about it before. He felt disorientated, excited, curious and unsure how to integrate these experiences into his current framework of being human. I explained that an electromagnetic field surrounds every organism and object in the Universe. They are often referred to as auras and can appear as shapes and colors. I offered other resources that could further explain what he saw. Many people are beginning to see, hear, or feel energy that was not readily accessible to them only a short time ago. These new perceptions are more common now. I was able to validate his experiences, which offered great relief to him. He continues exploring the larger field of consciousness.

Transformation can be messy, unclear, and uncomfortable. We can get too attached to a particular practice or become self-absorbed. If we get fixated on any one aspect of consciousness, it feeds the identification of **I am Individual,** and we can lose track of our intention to expand our awareness. We can get caught in judgment, excessive rumination, negative thinking and self-talk, and dysfunctional beliefs. Change does not occur without the discomfort and sacrifice of leaving old beliefs, meanings, and habits behind. Transformation takes intentional effort.

One of my clients was very involved with a particular Christian community. Her entire family's social and spiritual life was primarily limited to this group of people. She sang in the choir and was moved deeply by music. This led her to learning more about sound healing and chanting in other languages from different religious traditions. She began taking vacations without family members, attending workshops around the country, and studying with various teachers. Her family became upset, worried, and angry. They were not interested in understanding or supporting her growing passion. She felt rejected and abandoned. We were able to discuss her excitement, fear, pain, and joy as they arose throughout her transformation. She continued singing in the choir, and her enthusiasm delighted other parishioners. Eventually she was accepted back into her family as they realized she had not forsaken them or her religious community, but had expanded to include new paradigms and ways of expressing her Divine voice in the world. She transcended to a larger worldview, including all wisdom and compassion from her previous experiences.

Coaches invite us towards our inner capacity for healing, wisdom, and compassion. Coaches assist us in assimilating, integrating, and stabilizing higher consciousness, and can be invaluable on the journey. They remind us that our state of Holiness is always present, even if our focus is on our gaps or holes, making wholeness feel elusive.

Reflection

Are you involved in communities that support your journey towards higher consciousness?

Have you engaged with practitioners who have been encouraging and offered useful strategies for transformation? Are there supportive services you would like to explore?

Are there beneficial relationships you would like to find, nurture, or deepen that are supportive of your goals for transformation?

Have you experienced the transforming process as messy or uncomfortable at times?

What concentrative practices do you engage in when your attention is caught in repetitive thoughts and emotions focused on worry in the past or future?

What transforming practices do you use for self-exploration?

How could a transformational coach be beneficial in supporting you as you open your awareness to higher levels of consciousness?

CHAPTER NINE

CHANGING MINDS

Through our ability to direct our attention and expand our awareness, we can increase our capacity to function at higher levels of consciousness on a cellular level.

How does transformation to higher consciousness actually happen? Let's explore the process more deeply by examining how our perspectives, minds, and bodies shift as we move towards higher consciousness.

Modern insights and discoveries have shown us how our cells literally create, connect, and transform differently depending upon our level of calm or arousal. Through our ability to direct our attention and expand our awareness, we can increase our capacity to function at higher levels of consciousness on a cellular level. We know the dual nature of the wave-particle element means it changes from a waveform to a particle when it is observed. Similarly, the part of our brain that grows is determined by the focus of our attention. If we choose to focus on trauma or drama, we grow the part of our brains responsible for surviving. If we are calm and non-reactive, we grow the area of the brain that is responsible for complex reasoning and compassion.

In science classes many years ago, we were taught that a person does not grow new brain cells. However, recent research on the brain through advanced imaging technologies led to the discovery of neurogenesis, validating that the process of growing new brain cells is natural. The brain has the intrinsic ability to modify neural pathways and connections through changes in our behavior, thoughts, learning, and environment. This is called neuroplasticity. Old beliefs told us the brain was a static organ. Not true. We create circuits in our brain based on repetition of our thoughts and emotions. Our beliefs, paradigms, and viewpoints shift as we have access to more of the field of consciousness. These changes are mirrored in our brain cells.

So how do these changes in our brain support our transformation? The brain can be thought of as a control center of the body. We can imagine it is like a call center receptionist who answers incoming phone calls and sends outgoing messages all over the mind-body to their proper destination. Consider the brain in three regions, separated by location and function. They are the brainstem, the limbic system and the cortex. The brain is actually a much more sophisticated system, but this simplified explanation will help us explore its role and function related to expanding awareness and higher consciousness.

The brainstem houses our animal instincts and autonomic nervous system. The main function of this region is to keep us safe and help us stay alive. It was the first to develop and is responsible for balance and equilibrium, movement coordination, and autonomic functions such as breathing, heart rate, and digestion. If danger is detected, this region of the brain is activated and our instinct to survive kicks in. Our fight, flight, or freeze response is a wonderful protective mechanism when real threats are present. However, our brain has no discernment between real and imagined stimulus.

If the brainstem is turned on when no threat is actually present or if we worry about an imaginary threat, we stay trapped in the survival mode of lower level consciousness. This process creates more brain cells in this region and reinforces these connections.

The limbic system, relatively in the middle of the brainstem and frontal lobes, is a collection of separate structures that support functions such as emotion, motivation, learning, and long-term memory. This region of the brain receives and processes sensory information through our eyes, ears, thinking, and perceiving. It gives us the ability to feel and remember experiences. As we have new encounters, it is this processing center that lets us know if we are safe or unsafe by comparing it to previous experiences.

The cortex, in the front and outer parts of the brain, is responsible for attention, perceptual awareness, thought, writing, language, complex reasoning, problem solving, and perception of consciousness. This region houses our ability for higher order thinking, conscious thought, reflection, and selfless love. This area was the last to be developed in the evolution of the human brain, and is the section biologically programmable for bliss and extraordinary longevity. Growing more brain cells and connections in this region supports our ability to sustain higher levels of consciousness.

These three parts work together. Auditory and visual information is received and gets sorted through a region of the limbic system called the thalamus. The information gets relayed along two pathways simultaneously. One is a short pathway to the amygdala, a region of the limbic system. The second is a longer pathway to the cortex.

The amygdala processes emotions such as fear, anger, and pleasure, and stores memories. As a new sensory stimulus flashes through the amygdala, it determines if there are any matches to the information. It establishes if we are in a threatening situation or not. If perceived we are not safe, the brain automatically activates the fight, flight, or freeze response. Then, we only have access to our brainstem functions, which are instinctual and focused on survival. Often we have a strong emotional reaction which has a sudden onset. This can lead us to react irrationally and destructively. It creates more "fear" brain cells and circuits. When we feel unsafe, we avoid, protect, and withdraw. The pathway to the cortex and higher brain function is shut off.

If the amygdala verifies there is no threat by reviewing the stored memories relating to this sensory input, the second pathway to the cortex is completed. Here we process our incoming information with full access to our capacity for speech, higher order thinking, sensory perception, witness perspective, and cognizant thought. When input follows the path to the cortex, we are capable of responding instead of reacting, we are able to grow and expand instead of closing down. When we feel safe, we cultivate satisfaction and connection.

Transforming practices, designed to center us in the present moment quiet, still, and open the mind-body-heart help create conditions to activate higher brain functioning. We can interrupt the conditioned thalamus to amygdala to fight-flight reactivity when no danger actually exists in the present moment. We can literally grow new brain cells and create more active and connected neuropathways in the cortex which makes it easier to stay in the present moment. As we know, the brain is not infinitely plastic, but practices that lead to rewiring are very beneficial.

I learned about creating new brain cells and pathways years ago when I was working at a small clinic pharmacy and was held up at gunpoint. Two men carrying guns barreled in near closing time demanding the narcotics. I quickly took all of the drugs they wanted from the safe and dropped them in their athletic bag as ordered. They exited in a thunder, leaving my technician and me in a highly activated stress response. Shaking, sweating, heart pounding, nauseated, afraid and angry, I called 9-1-1. The robbers were never caught. I felt violated and betrayed.

During the months that followed, I began to notice uncontrollable sweating, shaking, fear, and heart racing for no apparent reason. Bringing my attention and witness observer to these episodes, I realized whenever I heard the sound of people running and coins or keys jingling unexpectedly, I was triggered into an all-out stress response. Then I remembered the connection. When the robbers rushing with guns pointed at me stormed into the pharmacy, they also had keys or coins jingling. With that sound trigger, my limbic system recognized that sensory input as danger. The new cells and pathways laid down in my hindbrain during that robbery were activated. Remember, the brain cannot tell the difference between an actual event occurring and one being imagined or recreated in some way. With this insight, I could begin the process of disconnecting that trigger to my stress response.

Whenever I heard the sound of feet pounding and coins jingling, I could feel the stress reaction and emotions begin. I brought all of my attention into the present moment, took a deep breath, and where possible took a few minutes for a deeper transforming practice like mindful walking, listening to music, or a meditation on peaceful imagery. I reminded myself from my witness perspective that in the present moment I was not in danger. The connection started to fade. Eventually the sound of coins jingling and people running caused no stress response, leaving only a neutral memory, which did not hook me into reactivity. Along with the rewiring of neural pathways came forgiveness and freedom from resentment and anger.

Every time we are able to notice ourselves over reacting to a sensory stimulus attached to an old memory, we have a choice. We can bring our attention into the present moment of safety and activate the relaxation response. Even disconnecting small associations like an aversion to a smell or sound or being hypervigilant in a certain place are beneficial. There may be topics of conversation that make us fly into rage or that we avoid because it knowingly or unknowingly reminds us of another time we felt unsafe. Old connections and brain cells cease if not reinforced by taking attention away from thought and emotion patterns that no longer serve our expanding consciousness. As we gently remove our attention from false drama and trauma, we heal our holes. Our reactivity fades over time, moving us closer to wholeness.

This process works in reverse when we focus our attention on cultivating higher brain functions.

Invitation to Practice

- Do certain visual or auditory input activate your stress response even though no danger is actually occurring in that present moment? When you notice the connection, work with transforming practices to calm your mind-body. Stop and do a practice every time you notice. This will unhook that false and automatic memory of danger from the triggers and free you from your conditioned reactivity.

- Notice a positive experience. Spend ten minutes reinforcing the feelings, memories, and gratitude that accompany this event. What are your insights? How can you increase your capacity to cultivate delight and joy in your life?

If we have a positive experience and have an emotional response that creates joy, satisfaction, or contentment, it is useful to stop and linger in this experience. Spend a few moments being grateful. Feel the physical sensations of being delighted.

Notice the connection to the source of pleasure. Maybe it is a person, nature, or an event that is being observed. When we stop and appreciate insights, it enhances our higher brain function and grows cortex brain cells and connectivity. This in turn increases our capacity to solve a complex problem, increases our sense of bliss and increases our capacity for selfless love. In short, it expands our perception and opens our awareness to a larger portion of the field of consciousness.

In addition to our brain cells changing, there are shifts in other cells that support evolution of consciousness. The health of our cells is influenced by the thoughts, feelings, and choices we experience moment to moment. As we discussed earlier, one area of the cell impacted by our stress and relaxation responses are the DNA. Deoxyribonucleic acid is present in every cell and are known as the blueprint of life. It contains the biological instructions needed to construct other components of cells. Stress produces chemicals and hormones that can turn off and on parts of our DNA called genomes, which can cause or prevent disease throughout our body. For instance, a healthy cell environment keeps cell growth in check and repairs damaged DNA. In addition, our bodies produce healthy chemicals when we relax that protect the end of our DNA called telomeres, which can lengthen a person's life span.

Enlightenment can be described as the condition of optimal mitochondrial and brain functioning. As we mentioned, mitochondria are components inside our cells that take the oxygen we breathe and the food we eat and process it to make energy, the fuel for life. Stress hormones are chemicals such as adrenaline, cortisol, norepinephrine, glucocorticoids, catecholamines, and vasopressin. They are involved in physiological process that can lead to decreased mitochondrial health and wear away telomeres. Eventually, the molecular decay and membrane injury of mitochondria and the erosion of telomeres can damage our DNA and lead to the death of cells. Healthy cells throughout the body allow us to experience both wellbeing and inner peace and the urge to create and innovate. Optimal cell health and brain function support higher consciousness.

This new knowledge reinforces the importance of adequate and balanced sleep, nutrition, supplements, stress reduction, and exercise. Oxidation, inflammation, and toxicity all lead to decreased cell health, not only in our brains but throughout our mind-body. In addition to managing our stress and cultivating calm in our mind-bodies, we can minimize toxins and inflammation by increasing antioxidants and phytonutrients from fresh vegetables, fruits, beans, nuts, seeds, and whole grains. When we eat phytonutrients (chemicals found in plants), they help prevent disease and keep our bodies working properly. Plants contain more than 100,000 phytonutrients, one of the reasons nine servings of fruits and vegetables a day are recommended. Some act as antioxidants in our bodies and tackle harmful free radicals that damage tissue throughout our bodies. Some may help protect against cancer by slowing down the growth of cancer cells and by helping our liver neutralize cancer-causing chemicals in our system. Examples of good sources of phytonutrients are greens such as spinach, kale and collards, strawberries, raspberries, dates, pomegranates, and green tea.

We can experiment with an elimination diet which involves removing specific foods or ingredients from our diet because they may be causing allergy symptoms or adverse effects. Common allergy-causing foods include milk, eggs, nuts, gluten, wheat, and soy. After eliminating or taking foods out of our diet, we can gradually reintroduce into our diet the foods we were avoiding. Add them one at a time over time. Notice which foods are causing inflammation, allergy symptoms, or adverse effects.

In addition, we could experiment by eliminating alcohol and sugar for a week and notice any changes in our body-mind. Sugar and alcohol help yeast and harmful bacteria in our gut thrive. Reducing heavily processed food can benefit our cell health also. They often contain high amounts of transfats, which raise our bad cholesterol while lowering our good. They usually contain excessive amounts of sugar. They often have large amounts of sodium, which can lead to increased blood pressure, which in turn contributes to heart disease and stroke. Some synthetic chemicals used in the processed foods industry are known to have carcinogenic properties. Examples of processed foods include crackers, sausage, and cheese sauce.

It is empowering to understand the choices we make in our reactivity and what we feed our bodies can support or diminish our movement towards higher consciousness. These new scientific discoveries and deeper understanding of our mind-body at a cellular level inspire us to make changes that positively impact our development.

Reflection

Is there sensory input that triggers your fight, freeze, or flight response that you can unhook and heal?

What are the current foods and supplements that support your transformation? Are there new nutritional habits you are willing to begin to improve your brain and cell health? Are there habits you are willing to limit?

What activities and practices do you engage in that grow new pathways of higher brain function and cells in your cortex?

PART THREE

THE LIGHT: BEING HOLY

CHAPTER TEN

LIVING INTERCONNECTED

*When we live a life as **I am Interconnected** we are mystics seeing the unifying vision of the One in the All and the All in the One.*

The fulfillment of **I am Individual** yields a productive and contributing citizen capable of meaningful relationships and feelings of purpose, self-confidence, passion, and self-worth. This self-actualizing person can live freely without fear, and do what he or she intends to in the world in a reasonably well-harmonized way. It would be amazing if all human beings fully functioned at this level of consciousness, and if our social institutions supported such full functioning.

As we yearn for more, we continue expanding our awareness, living with a wider view and seeing ourselves as part of the sea of consciousness rather than separate from it. What does full embodiment of **I am Interconnected** look like? We recognize thoughts, feelings, and body sensations often connected to occurrences outside of our personal self. Our ability to innovate, create, and find abundance is readily accessible.

We participate in service through focusing our intention and moving toward aligned co-creative opportunities. Seemingly miraculous people or circumstances arise in our lives that are the perfect fit of complementary skills and resources. We contribute by knowing and utilizing our talents and passions. Focusing on only our personal gain is replaced by being a humanitarian and focusing on the good of the whole, including ourselves.

Another word for living a life as **I am Interconnected** is a mystic. We see the unifying vision of the One in the All and the All in the One. Once we have an experience of unity, our worldview is forever shifted. There is no longer an experience of "other" as disconnected from ourselves. The interconnection of self and other remains in our awareness. There are many names for mystics; saints originated in Christianity, the Jewish name is Tzadik, the Islamic Mu'min, the Hindu Rishi, and the Buddhist arhat or bodhisattva. Mystics recognize a sense of oneness, wholeness and completeness. We experience a feeling of encountering what some call the "the true self," a sense of the nature of our essential cosmic self. This self is beyond life and death, beyond difference and duality, and beyond ego and selfishness.

The witness observer softens and relaxes, expanding our perspective to see connection and information from the once apparently invisible realm of subtle energies and vibrations throughout the sea of consciousness. We often receive more frequent intuitive and inspiring knowing. Daily occurrences more often appear miraculous, strokes of genius, and ecstatic. Joy can be experienced for no apparent reason, not requiring an external or internal trigger.

Additional characteristics of **I am Interconnected** include aligning with the flow, revelation, paradox, and synchronicity. These experiences become more accessible and provide regular information useful in daily living. Because we have the capacity to maintain a still centered mind-body, we have free attention to notice, sense, and experience subtle levels of energy that occur continuously. Our experience of being in the flow in lower consciousness is often a random occurrence, without any realization of where it came from or why it leaves. At this heightened level of consciousness, we can focus our attention and intention and align our self with the flow, creating access to the uplifting sensations of bliss, full engagement, and expansion that characterize this way of knowing. This identification of being human is marked by such qualities as tolerance, unity, trust, joy, ease, and peacefulness. Cooperation and collaboration, energy awareness, connection to the natural world and intuition are common. Embodying this level of consciousness is a gift to ourselves and all beings.

When we live as **I am Interconnected**, we are often creative, fresh, alive, and prolific and can manifest in expressions such as a sage, mystic, artist, teacher, inventor, or healer. Living as this full expression is a way of being in the world no matter what activity we are doing.

Meister Eckhart reminds us it is who we are, not what we do, that matters the most:

> People ought not to consider so much what they are to do as what they are; let them but be good and their ways and deeds will shine brightly. If you are just, your actions will

be just too. Do not think that saintliness comes from occupation; it depends rather on what one is. The kind of work we do does not make us Holy, but we may make it Holy. However "sacred" a calling may be, as it is a calling, it has no power to sanctify; but rather as we are and have the divine being within, we bless each task we do, be it eating, or sleeping, or watching, or any other.[13]

Paradox replaces the tightly held beliefs and perspective of opposites such as right and wrong, good and bad, light and dark, in and out, East and West, warm and cold, and yours and mine. These become descriptors on a continuum of experience. When does east become west? Or hot become cold? That meaning is applied depending on our current perspective. In Minnesota where I live, after the cold winter months, 54°F can feel warm and inviting. At the end of summer, 54°F can feel chilly and uninviting. When we see the continuum, we step back and see the whole range of possibilities. We still utilize discernment, but we do not infuse what is with judgment and false meaning.

In paradox, ideas may seem to contradict each other yet all be true simultaneously. Other times we can know something to be true and untrue at the same time. We embrace paradox when we have the ability to realize contradiction and both sides of an issue. We transcend the limits of logical reasoning. We can be detached and fully present (here and now) in the drama of life. We can be self-disciplined, yet act in a spontaneous manner at times. We can have an experience filled with many contradicting emotions.

---

13. Meister Eckhart, *Christian Social Teachings: A Reader in Christian Social Ethics from the Bible to the Present* (Minneapolis: Fortress Press, 2013), 71.

When I left my full-time corporate job, I was incredibly frightened and excited at the same time. I had no plan for my next job, yet I trusted it would appear with my attention and intention contributing to what was occurring. As pointed out, paradox may be at odds with the current norms of society. Paradox can produce cognitive dissonance which is a feeling of uncomfortable tension, which comes from holding two conflicting thoughts in the mind at the same time. As our awareness of the world grows, often our experience reveals contradictions with the traditions we were taught. This presents us with a paradox which is a normal aspect of our growth in consciousness.

We can discern good from bad, yet go beyond both. We cultivate compassion and relieve suffering, and also accept that everything is perfect just the way it is. We have discussed the paradox at the quantum level where a particle exists in a suspended state, a sort of super-animation, until it is actually observed. At the point of observation, it takes on the form of either a particle or wave, while still having the properties of both. We experience paradox when we see ourselves as separate bodies and personalities, but we are also indivisible parts of the Whole. Metaphorically we are individual waves which rise and fall on the one great ocean of Being, with which our higher identity is linked.

Intuition flourishes in a person who is open, receptive, discerning, and nonjudgmental. It is a capacity we all possess. Intuitive information is neutral, and the more we practice paying attention the more familiar we become with the subtle vibration of intuitive knowing and the more clearly we can interpret it. Answers to lightly held questions and insights can come in a song you hear on the radio, a seemingly random encounter or event, a knowing or sensation in your body, images in your mind's eye, a feeling, or an inner voice. Often answers come unexpectedly while you go about your daily activities and routine. Remember intuition is non-local; it transcends and contains time and space.

Here is an example of the practical application of intuition. One Saturday, I spent the day doing chores and errands. I wandered from doing dishes, to sorting the mail, to folding laundry. I had done a few errands in the morning and midday was heading out again, which prompted my rituals of brushing my teeth and putting on a ring I frequently wore. I could not find my ring. I started to retrace my steps since I had returned. My left brain was activated, that part that is logical, sequential, rational, analytical, objective and looks at the parts and pieces. I remembered wearing it out for my morning errands. After I returned, I did the dishes. My routine is to put my ring in my pants pocket or night-stand when not wearing it. I was not wearing pants that had pockets and it was not in my nightstand. I headed out with freshly brushed teeth and no ring. Maybe its whereabouts would come to me.

When I returned, I carefully looked in the kitchen, by the desk, and in the laundry room. My stress response was starting; I could feel myself becoming anxious, my heart beat increasing, slight sweating on the palm of my hands, and the clouding of my thoughts. All of my logical thinking and looking did not produce a ring. I knew for certain it was somewhere in the house. It was time to tap into another way of knowing, my intuition, and intentionally activate my right brain. This part of our brain is intuitive, holistic, synthesizing, subjective, and looks at the whole. I sat down, shut my eyes, and got very quiet in my mind and body. I took a few deep breaths and centered all of my attention in the present moment. Out of the stillness an image of complete blackness emerged in my mind's eye. As I continued to breathe, I could expand my view of this darkness. As I did, a bit of light came into my vision and I saw a pile of something. Still uncertain of the images I was seeing, I relaxed further and the screen in my mind's eye expanded. It was the garbage can in the kitchen. I got up, dug through the layers of mail I had tossed earlier, and found my ring at the bottom.

Relieved, I retraced the steps of my day again and re-engaged my logical left brain ways of knowing. A pocket in my pants was unavailable, but I was wearing a jean shirt with a pocket in the top left corner where I placed my ring before starting the dishes. While sorting the mail I had tossed it off the desk onto the hallway floor into a big pile, then scooped it up and put it in the garbage. The ring had fallen out of my shirt pocket into the pile which I put into the garbage can in the kitchen. I was filled with gratitude for asking for help, the assistance I received, and the practical application of intuition. With just my five senses, I would not have found that ring.

Since that experience, initiated by utter despair and surrender, I continue to cultivate my intuition. Pictures in my mind's eye, sounds, words, physical sensations in my body, thoughts, feelings, and even a sense of smell and taste may come as I turn my attention to my intuitive way of knowing. It has become

more accessible and continues to be very practical in my work
with clients and daily living.

Invitation to Practice

- Find a time when you are completely relaxed. Maybe
before you enter your morning shower. Maybe a
morning when you are waking up refreshed with no
pressing commitment requiring you to get out of bed
right away. When you are already relaxed it is easier to access an even wider perspective in the sea of
consciousness.

- Take a moment to recall an intention you have for
more clarity. Maybe it is on a decision you are contemplating. Maybe you are looking for deeper insight
into a pattern you realize causes suffering in your
life. Gently bring your intention to mind.

- Continue your relaxed state of being for another
few minutes. Feel your intention with all five senses.
Invite your intuition and other ways of knowing into
your awareness. With open non-judgmental awareness, rest your attention in the present moment.

- Notice if any wisdom arises that provides clarity.
Spend a few minutes in gratitude.

I smile as I recall my daughter calling from college in
California years later to ask for assistance. She had lost her access
card which tracked her meal plan and was used to get in and out
of buildings on campus. A picture emerged in my mind with her

request to help find it. I saw her using her access card as a book-mark, and it had slid into the pages of the book. As she walked around her apartment, telling me about her English class lecture that day and the party the night before with her friends, I could hear the book pages fanning in the background. Eventually the access card dropped out of one. She thanked me and continued sharing her stories. I smile with a grateful heart knowing my children find intuition an ordinary and reliable way of knowing.

Living with access to intuition further attunes us to the higher and more subtle vibrations around us, in us, and between us. With this access, creativity is amplified. Deeper understanding of self and other is revealed. Living as **I am Interconnected,** we become more tolerant, accepting and loving towards others and ourselves as the realization that we are all interconnected expands. Intuition is an amazing line of communication with the sea of consciousness.

Another characteristic of this level of consciousness is synchronicity or meaningful coincidence. This is the coming together of inner and outer events in a way that cannot be explained by cause and effect yet is significant to us. Our minds have the amazing ability to relate events and phenomena that may seem unrelated to one another. Noticing recurring words, colors, objects, stories, or animals are a wonderful example of synchronicity. Perceiving and knowing through symbols that appear in our inner and outer life can provide powerful information, knowledge and wisdom.

I had a client who was in a transition personally and professionally. She was going through a divorce, moving and making a career change. Dragonflies began to appear. She was staying with a friend who had a dragonfly shower curtain. She received an invitation to a birthday party with a dragonfly pin on the front. Another friend gave her a silk dragonfly scarf, and her sister sent her a card with a beautiful hand-painted dragonfly.

During a session we looked up the symbolic meaning of dragonflies in a variety of places. Among many interesting insights into the meaning of dragonflies, we discovered that dragonflies may symbolize coming into a two-year period of transformation. They may reflect a need to institute changes that may culminate in the colorful transformations we desire. The appearance of dragonflies assured her she was exactly where she needed to be and allowed her to further relax into her experience. Once she settled into her new home and career, the dragonflies no longer appeared. The entire process of transition was about two years.

Reflection

What are some of your stories of events that occurred in amazing and synergistic timing that provide a revelation, inspiration, or delight in your life?

How do you cultivate intuition?

What synchronicities have you noticed that have given you insight?

Describe a paradox you have become aware of. Did it affect your thoughts, feeling, or the way you live?

CHAPTER ELEVEN

RADIATING ESSENCE

When we are reduced to the merest point, a speck of identity closing the last minuscule gap between ourselves and God, we have realized our **Center Within.**

Living reliably in the stage of middle consciousness, **I am Interconnected**, allows a tremendous amount of freedom. Self-awareness in the present moment is consistently available, giving us the choice to respond rather than react out of unrealized conditioned habits. Through dependable alignment with the flow and access to the sea of consciousness, we live knowing we have everything we need in every moment. Continuing our natural tendency to ever-expanding levels for consciousness, we gain even more freedom.

When we experience ourselves as **I am Infinite** and subject and object merge into one identity, there is another quantum leap in perspective. Pure awareness lives as the expression of form in the world, shifting moment to moment. Our primary identity at this level of consciousness is that which remains unchanging, the Ground of Being from which all springs forth, instead of that which is continuously changing. In Hinduism, this feeling that one has encountered the true self is expressed in the idea that ātman (the individual self) and Brahman (the cosmic self: literally, the breath [brah] of the universe) are one and the same. We experience the manifest and unmanifest world as an expression of pure essence. We realize our true inner nature that has always been present as ourselves.

Invitation to Practice

- Take three deep breaths, in through your nose and out through your mouth. Feel your belly soften as it expands and contracts.

- Scan your body. Breathe into any part that feels tight or sore. Relax fully.

- Imagine a peaceful place. It could be a place you vacation, a place in nature, or your home. Allow the sights, sounds, smells, and feel of this peace filled place relax you even more deeply.

- Imagine a time you have been lost in the pleasure of an experience. Your joy in the moment was so complete you did not realize time passing. You were immersed in the bliss of the moment. Allow the sensations of that moment to radiate throughout your being.

- When you are ready, bring your attention back to your breath.

- Set aside 30 minutes a week to engage in an activity you enjoy just for the sake of delight, with no particular purpose to be productive or recognized.

This experience of higher consciousness may occur when we have been completely absorbed in an activity. We have mentioned behaviors such as gardening or running where there is just oneness; not even a doer and the doing or seer and seeing. This is also the condition during deep dreamless sleep where there is no activity or event happening, just undifferentiated pure awareness. We have noted another time we may recognize this condition of unity is during lovemaking where there is no perception of where "I" end and "my beloved" begins.

While contemplating this sense of no subject or object, the picture that arose in my mind's eye is a submarine. In order for a submarine to navigate, it utilizes a sonar system which sends out a sound, a ping, that bounces off another object to inform it when to turn. It chooses the best route of navigation based on avoiding hazards and moving toward open spaces. In lower levels of consciousness, we often make choices to avoid pain or move toward pleasure. Imagine life if you sent out a ping and it never bounced off anything because everything that is, is you.

Your entire way of knowing yourself, the other, the interconnectedness of all things ceases and a new way of being and knowing arises. Every level of reality of a cell has its own relationships and laws which govern existence while being a part of many more encompassing levels. Likewise, **I am Infinite** is unique.

When we experience ourselves as **I am Infinite**, we have the unique viewpoint of experiencing infinity and the perception of infinite space without losing our sense of individuality. We experience all levels of consciousness simultaneously. There is a paradoxical blend of universality and individuality. We transcend paradox and know every level of reality is a holographic experience. At every level, the micro and the macro are reflections of the one.

The Chandogya Upanishad (Volumes 2 through 7 of the second Prapathaka) teaches that:

> Everything in the entire universe—heaven, earth, and beyond—is contained in a small space within the heart: In this body, in this town of Spirit, there is a little house shaped like a lotus and in that house there is a little space. There is as much in that little space within the heart as there is in the whole world outside. Heaven, earth, fire, wind, sun, moon, lightning, stars; whatever is and whatever is not, everything is there.[14]

We live with a sense of being awake and in continuous balance. All of our attention is in the present moment; thus the past and future are also in this now. There is a sense of causeless joy, and a deep knowing of and trust in what is. Desire and choice give way as our awareness experiences every moment as unique. We live in the world like a dancer responding to music that calls us to move. Our identity rests in I AM, versus previous attachment to I am this or I am that. All of our unique qualities, preferences, and lineage continue to exist in and as us, but our primary identity rests in I AM. This condition has also been described as perfection, continually perfecting itself. Unity consciousness prevails.

---

14. Ānandagiri, Śaṅkarācārya, Jīvānanda Vidyāsāgara Bhaṭṭācāryya, *The Chandogya Upanishad of the Samaveda* (Sucharoo Press, 1873).

This level of consciousness is known by many names. It is sometimes called Presence, Atman, Suchness, God, The Void, Immovable Mover, All That Is, and The Omega Point. There are many qualities assigned to this level of consciousness such as infinite, eternal, omnipotence, omniscience, liberation, grace, heaven, paradise, awakening, enlightenment, transcendence, samadhi, mukti, satori, and nirvana. Living in this condition provides sensations of peace, serenity, calm, stillness, and purity. A Sufi poet, Baba Kuhi of Shiraz (d. 1050 CE), wrote:

> I opened mine eyes and by the light of His face around me
> In all the eye discovered – only God I saw.
> Like a candle I was melting in His fire:
> Amidst the flames outflanking – only God I saw.
> Myself with mine own eyes I saw most clearly,
> But when I looked away into nothingness, I vanished,
> And lo, I was the All-living – only God I saw.[15]

We recognize the world as a projection from the infinite unmanifested potential of the entire field of consciousness. This projection is nothing more than a point of view that comes to life. The highest point of view encompasses anything that happens without rejection. In this condition, we know all things and no thing at the same time. The Chinese called it the Tao, meaning the offstage presence that gives the world life, shape, purpose, and flow:

---

15. Reynold A. Nicholson, *The Mystics of Islam* (Sacramento: Murine Press, 2006), 23.

Two impossible things must converge. We are reduced to the merest point, a speck of identity closing the last minuscule gap between ourselves and God. [Here we have realized our **Center Within**.] At the same time, just when separation is healed, the tiny point expands to infinity. The mystics describe this as "the One becomes the All." To put it into quantum physics scientific terms, when we cross into the quantum zone, space-time collapses into itself. The tiniest thing in existence merges with the greatest; the point and infinity are equal.[16]

Any and all genuine practice can lead us to experience this state of consciousness, and for some their initial taste is a momentary state of bliss. We no longer experience a sense of practicing a technique as it becomes embodied at the fullest capacity. Practice becomes what is and disappears, along with all sense of separation. Transforming practices, the witness observer and service cease being activities and become embedded as a way of living moment to moment, a natural outpouring of expression with every breath. We become the flow, and life's activities arise from within as a response to present moment conditions and knowing. Our ability to live as the infinite eternal expression of All That Is becomes more stable and accessible each moment you know yourself as **I am Infinite**. You embody the teaching from the Bible, Psalm 46:10, be still and know that you are God. We shift from a perspective of being whole to being Holy.

T.S. Elliot, a 20th century poet, reminds us in his Four Quartets Section V writings that the world remains the same; it

---

16. Deepak Chopra, *How to Know God: The Soul's Journey into the Mystery of the Mysteries* (New York: Harmony Books, 2000), 96.

is our worldview that radically shifts as we transform our identity to **I am Infinite**:

> We shall not cease from exploration
> And the end of all our exploring
> Will be to arrive where we started
> And know the place for the first time.
> Through the unknown, unremembered gate
> When the last of earth left to discover
> Is that which was the beginning;
> At the source of the longest river
> The voice of the hidden waterfall
> And the children in the apple-tree
> Not known, because not looked for
> But heard, half-heard, in the stillness
> Between two waves of the sea.
> Quick now, here, now, always.
> A condition of complete simplicity
> (Costing not less than everything)
> And all shall be well and
> All manner of thing shall be well
> When the tongues of flame are in-folded
> Into the crowned knot of fire
> And the fire and the rose are one.[17]

17   T.S. Elliot, *Four Quartets* (Orlando: Houghton Mifflin Harcourt, 1943), 59.

Reflection

Are there readings or activities that open you into knowing yourself as **I am Infinite**?

Do you recognize resistance or beliefs in yourself, in the people around you, or in society that make it feel difficult to know yourself as Holy?

What would it be like to live an entire hour with the freedom of continual acceptance that you are perfection continually perfecting itself? How would you feel in that state of being?

PART FOUR

THE WORLD: EVERYDAY MYSTIC

CHAPTER TWELVE

RELATING FROM YOUR CENTER WITHIN

When we embody higher consciousness, we call each other forward to live as our whole and Holy selves.

Once we have tasted the sweet joy and peace of **I am Infinite** and know ourselves as the essence of All That Is, our worldview is radically, irreversibly, and forever changed. When we feel unity, there is no longer an experience of an "other" someone or something as disconnected from ourselves. The interconnection of self and other remains in our awareness.

This perspective profoundly impacts our relationships. When we deeply see another person, we recognize our identical inner nature. We honor and salute the love shining from the core of all beings. We respect each person's journey and chosen pace as we move toward discovering our essence of Holiness. We realize it would be unloving to impose our worldview on another. With discernment, we recognize each relationship is unique and engage accordingly. Right action and right relationship arise in present moment awareness.

We may discern all kinds of differences in our expression of Divine nature, but that does not occlude our knowing that we share one core essence. Often there are parts of ourselves and others, inside and outside, which are still not whole. In any given moment we may slip back into **I am Individual**, feeling the holes of separation. Since we have experienced unity, we are more likely to be kinder and gentler when this condition arises. We may approach our self and one another as we would a puppy or a child when we notice suffering. We do not accept bad behavior, violence, or others imposing immature ideals. We are moved to heal the wounds of separation in our own mind-body and in our relationships with an open heart.

Our relationships mirror our level of consciousness. When we live in lower consciousness and are primarily focused on healing our holes, we see each person as autonomous. From this viewpoint, we often see the other as the source of our suffering and happiness. We tend to blame them for not bringing us enough joy and for causing us pain. In our conversations, we can be defensive, need to impose our opinions as the only right idea on the other, and feel like a victim. We may recognize patterns of dissatisfaction and discontentment. We may move from job to job or relationship to relationship. At first there is excitement in the new relationship, then the inevitable complaining and judgement that our bosses and lovers are inadequate. Love is conditional. We are only able to love another if they are bringing us pleasure. We are seeking wholeness outside. The lessons will repeat indefinitely until we decide to heal our holes and find wholeness inside.

If, however, only one person is invested in developing more self-awareness and shifting to access a larger portion of the field of consciousness, incoherence can become intolerable for both people. As our understanding of who we are grows and changes, there can be sadness as we outgrow long-time relationships. We may lose interest in activities and ideas that we held in common. As our level of awareness grows, we may find less and less in common with people attached to their holes. As we embody mindful awareness, we often find it boring or distracting to engage in drama, gossip, or trauma. This can lead to a choice to move on from the relationship, or settle for connecting on a superficial level only. We can find ourselves longing for deeper connection while grieving the loss of old relationships. Other established relationships transform and grow with us as we become more vulnerable, real, and intimate.

When we are engaged in trusting relationships and are committed to practicing our own self-awareness, it is not necessary to be at the same level of consciousness. I remember a time when my daughter was in high school and decided to stay out way past her midnight curfew without checking in. By 12:30, I was livid. By 1:30, I was terrified. This was highly unusual. It was before the era of cell phones. I felt helpless and afraid. She strolled in around 2 AM. I greeted her with an explosion of relief, anger, and exhaustion. I had enough sense to tell her we would talk in the morning.

Her morning came sometime in the early afternoon. I was refreshed, calm, and open to listening to what had occurred the previous night. I was curious about her process for deciding to violate curfew without a word of discussion or calling. After she had a bite to eat and was awake and relaxed, we sat down to converse.

I began by telling her, "When you did not come home by midnight as is our agreed upon curfew, I was worried and felt angry, confused, and afraid. I expect you to be home by midnight or call if there is an extenuating circumstance."

She replied, "You are the most unreasonable mean mom ever! No one else at my high school has such a ridiculously early curfew!"

I could feel my jaw clench and my frustration arise. I took a deep breath and asked a question. "Not one other person at your high school has a curfew of midnight?" I knew, of course, several of her friends had the same curfew.

"Hardly any," was her response.

I waited. She went on to say that the previous evening was a special party. Her soccer team, where she was the captain, had won a big game, and they were celebrating at someone's house.

"Why didn't you ask permission for an exception to your curfew?" She answered by telling me I am generally inflexible and have a history of not listening to her point of view, so she decided not to risk asking and being declined. She went on to say it was very important for her to be there until the party ended, and she would have been embarrassed leaving early, so she decided to suffer the consequences instead of asking for permission to be out beyond curfew.

I was listening and could feel her sincerity. I summarized what she had said, validating her experience of feeling nervous, hesitant, and torn about asking for permission before she went out. Even if I did not agree with her, I could understand her perspective.

"Is there more?" I asked.

She relaxed, softened, and opened further. She reminded me she really likes to sleep, and often at the end of a long day of school and sports, having the excuse to be home at midnight due to her curfew is great because she is tired. She apologized for not being home on time, not calling, and for making me feel afraid and angry. She actually had heard me. We agreed to talk and listen with open hearts when these exceptional late night opportunities arise in the future. We both felt heard; we both felt loved. Being listened to is so closely connected to being loved that most of us feel they are one in the same. In the sacred space created in authentic relationships, we call each other forward towards higher consciousness.

A powerful transforming practice in relationships is deep listening. In my coaching practice, I speak of this so often I have made business cards with the key points of authentic communication. One side lists the steps of authentic listening:

- **Mirror:** *What I am hearing you say is...* Is this right? Is there more?
- **Summarize the essence:** Include experience, feelings, impact and request.
- **Validation:** I can understand your perspective... It makes sense because...

www.centerwithin.com

the Center Within

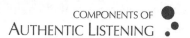
COMPONENTS OF
AUTHENTIC LISTENING

Actively listening in this way creates time and space for the other person to be heard and understood, letting him or her know his or her experience (and therefore person) matters. Deep listening reminds the listener of his or her connection to the speaker, moving us out of **I am Individual** into **I am Interconnected** and beyond. When we are authentically listening, we do not have to agree, just understand and validate the other person. In addition, both people conversing do not have to be engaged in authentic communication. If we have the ability to deeply listen, even if the other person is blaming, judging, or defending, this transforming practice of being heard usually deescalates the speaker and brings him or her back to calm. From this point of connection, we can move into productive conversation.

My communication cards are informed by Marshall Rosenberg's 4-part Nonviolent Communication process. His work is designed to help people to exchange the information necessary to resolve conflicts and differences with more ease, learn to ask for what a person wants without using demands, and begin to hear the true needs of others with less effort.

The other half of authentic communication is clear speaking. Use "I" statements instead of "you" statements. Speak about your own experience. When we use the word "you" instead of speaking about ourselves, it often sounds blaming and judging which automatically puts your listener on the defensive. I statements enhance the likelihood of being heard and having successful tender conversations and conflict resolution. On the other side of my authentic communication card is authentic speaking.

> ● **This is what I experienced.**
>
> ● **This was the impact on me, including feelings.**
>
> ● **This is what I want.**

www.centerwithin.com

the Center Within

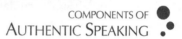
COMPONENTS OF ●
AUTHENTIC SPEAKING

When you start with what you experienced, make it neutral and factual. No embellishment or judgment. Just the facts. Be thoughtful about the impact this event or behavior had on you, and be sure to include your feelings. Many of us are not very skilled at recognizing and naming feelings. Own and express clearly the affect this experience had on you. Finally, be thoughtful with what you want. Be specific. Propose a solution to prevent this from occurring in the same way next time. When I spoke to my daughter about her late night out, I said, "When you did not come home by midnight as is our agreed upon curfew, I was worried and felt angry, confused and afraid. I expect you to be home by midnight or call if there is an extenuating circumstance."

- This is what I experienced: When you did not come home by midnight as is our agreed upon curfew.

- This was the impact it had on me including feelings: I was worried and felt angry, confused, and afraid.

- This is what I want: I expect you to be home by midnight or call if there is an extenuating circumstance.

In conflict, we often have the goal of getting the other person to accept or agree with our point of view. A critical part of conflict resolution is to change our goal from agreement to understanding. This is done through authentic communication.

The ageless wisdom of Mewlana Jalaluddin Rumi, 13th century Persian poet, Islamic scholar, theologian, and Sufi mystic, invites us to be in relationship in a field even beyond words:

> Out beyond ideas of wrongdoing and rightdoing,
> there is a field. I'll meet you there.
>
> When the soul lies down in that grass,
> the world is too full to talk about.
> Ideas, language, even the phrase "each other"
> doesn't make any sense.[18]

When we embody higher consciousness, our holes are whole so we are no longer searching to have our needs met by something or someone outside of ourselves. New relationships form with others giving attention and intention to healing holes, becoming whole and being Holy. We seek out and nurture mutually beneficial relationships and they become our norm. In conversations, we can act as a clear mirror, a witness observer, listening deeply and feeling our connection. We encourage each other to live from our passions, brilliance, and genius. We call

---

18.   Mewlana Jalaluddin Rumi, trans. Coleman Barks, *The Essential Rumi* (New York: Harper Collins Publishers, 1995), 16.

each other forward to live as our whole and Holy selves. Living in higher consciousness, we can be presence in our relationships, radiating a sense of ease and grace. We are able to be with others, hear them, and validate their experiences without any need to fix, change, or impose. Love is unconditional.

Invitation to Practice

- Find a place to relax for a few minutes. Take three deep breaths in and out. Feel your body soften.

- Invite a tender or conflict-resolving conversation you would like to have with someone who matters in your life to arise in your awareness.

- Take time to reflect:

  › What actually happened that has caused you to remain unsettled?

  › How did this incident make you feel?

  › What impact did this circumstance have on your body, heart, life?

  › If you could resolve this tender issue or conflict, what is the outcome you desire?

- When you are ready, write down what you would say to this person to work towards healing the sense of separation and misunderstanding.

- Find uninterrupted time to create sacred space and dialogue utilizing authentic communication.

In authentic relationships where both people are continuously and intentionally expanding awareness, gathering attention, clarifying intentions, and exploring what it means to cultivate openings to higher consciousness, we can be a mirror for each other. If one person gets stressed, reactive, complains, gossips or blames, the other can observe without judgment and reflect back what he or she notices. The person witnessing can acknowledge their partner's thoughts, feelings and reactions. He or she can invite the reactive partner to bring the focus back to him or herself. The partner embodying the highest level of consciousness in the moment can hold the vision of the other as complete, whole, and Holy until the other is able to claim it.

In chapter six I shared a story about my billing center manager being a mirror to me. She was a master of witnessing when she observed my hostility during the meeting we were attending. She summarized and validated my feelings of impatience and frustration. In addition, she challenged me to be kind as well as right. We had a respectful relationship built on numerous occasions where we had debated, listened, and resolved issues. Her ability to be my witness that day elevated my capacity to live interconnected. When we engage in these transparent vulnerable relationships, our access to higher consciousness can be accelerated.

Anthony de Mello reminds us how to love in relationship:

The first act of love is to see this person or this object, this reality as it truly is.

And this involves the enormous discipline of dropping your desires, your prejudices, your memories, your projections, your selective way of looking...a discipline so great that most people would rather plunge headlong into good actions and service than submit to the burning fire of this asceticism. When you set out to serve someone whom you have not taken the trouble to see, are you meeting that person's need or your own?[19]

In addition to authentic relationships, we stay engaged in practicing self-awareness. When we see ourselves being disappointed and reactive, we have an opportunity to heal our own holes. In chapter six I told a story about being upset with a bank teller. If I had been able to see the bank teller as performing her task in the best way possible, maybe I would not have slammed my cup of water down so hard. Maybe if I had noticed my pulse racing, my teeth clenching, my hands sweating or my son slithering towards the door utterly embarrassed, I would have stopped and spent a few minutes engaging in a transforming practice. Maybe I could have found the equanimity, the capacity to be mentally and emotionally stable and composed under tension, instead of being engulfed in my rage.

There is a timeless teaching from the Sufi tradition on the value of authentic speaking:

Before you speak, let your words pass through three gates.
At the first gate, ask yourself, 'Is it true?'
At the second ask, 'Is it necessary?'
At the third gate ask 'Is it kind?'[20]

19. Anthony de Mello, *Anthony De Mello: Writings* (New York: Orbis Books, 1999), 132.

20. Ben-Ami Scharfstein, *Mystical Experience* (Indianapolis: Bobbs-Merrill, 1973).

The recent discovery of mirror neurons adds to our understanding of the importance of relationships. Mirror neuron cells present in various cortex regions of the brain are activated both when we perform an action and when we watch another person perform the same action. They make our brains act as if we ourselves were experiencing whatever the other person is experiencing. This neural mechanism is involuntary and automatic. With it, we don't have to think about what other people are doing or feeling, we simply know. It is our neurological Wi-Fi.

These neurons are part of the process of experiencing empathy, the ability to share someone else's feelings. They are also involved in learning language and imitation. Both empathy and language are important in relationships. This evidence further illustrates the value of self-regulating and increasing our capacity to stay calm, open, and present like the wise Chinese farmer in chapter six. We are continuously attuning to the resonance of each other's nervous system. It is important to develop the capacity to maintain our higher consciousness and not mirror another's nervous system that is more aroused or reactive than our own.

The new field of interpersonal neurobiology reminds us that the brain is constantly rewiring itself based on daily life, which includes our relationships. What we pay the most attention to defines us. Our closest relationships that foster us or fail us alter the delicate circuits that shape memories, emotions and our self. Whether we feel heard and understood or not influences how genes express themselves and remodels the brain's architecture and functions. For instance, if we are in a healthy relationship, holding our partner's hand is enough to subdue our blood pressure, ease our response to stress, improve our health and soften physical pain. We alter one another's physiology and neural functions.

Have you noticed during a quickly deteriorating argument that you and your opponent can become illogical? Unable to process another's point of view? Unable to problem solve and be reasonable? If you both escalate to assessing the situation as dangerous and need to go into protection mode, you do not have access to the cortex area of your brain responsible for reflection, complex reasoning, problem solving, and higher order thinking. There is much wisdom in the old advice to count to ten, take a break, or breathe deeply to calm down and revisit the issue later.

If we cannot keep our mind-body relaxed, our limbic system will only allow processing in the brainstem and we will remain on high alert with our fight, flight or freeze stress response turned on. We are all invited to continue our evolution towards higher consciousness and increase activity in the cortex by cultivating a mind-body that is healthy, relaxed, still, and at peace in our relationships. This is especially true when we engage in tender conversations or conflict.

Communication modalities are changing and becoming more accessible every day. We have opportunities to build relationships with people via chat rooms, Twitter, instant messaging, email, Skype, and Facetime. It is important to build our communication skills and understand our many layers of interconnectedness. Now is the time for co-creating new solutions, structures, paradigms, stories about who are and what we value. Relating to each other from our **Center Within** at higher levels of consciousness contributes to our capacity to form new systems to better serve humanity.

Reflection

Is there a person in your life who is an authentic witness for you? How has this accelerated your growth? Facilitated your wholeness? Expanded your awareness?

Name a person you admire for his or her developed capacity to deeply listen and clearly speak. What qualities does he or she demonstrate that you would like to emulate?

Do you have long standing relationships that have changed as you have expanded your awareness and level of consciousness? Have some become more authentic and trusting? Are there some that have become more difficult, boring, or distracting?

How can you cultivate your capacity to authentically speak and listen in your relationships?

CHAPTER THIRTEEN

CONTRIBUTING FROM YOUR CENTER WITHIN

*When we live as our whole and Holy self, we radiate
our passion and catalyze transformation.*

Our level of consciousness ripples out beyond our self to our families, communities, organizations, the planet and the collective. When we know ourselves to be **I am Interconnected** or **I am Infinite**, we contribute to the many groups we participate in through our worldview of embodied wholeness and holiness. By our example in families, volunteer teams, communities, and work groups we encourage creativity, passion, productivity, balance, cohesion, and authenticity. This creates the conditions for amazing new paradigms and solutions that encourage our collective good to manifest.

The need to contribute is inherent in each of us. We are hardwired to connect and are driven by an internal sense of reward when we bond with others. Our brains secrete a hormone called oxytocin, which is sometimes known as the cuddle hormone. It plays a role in processing social information we receive such as sights, touch, and sound and links our experience to the brain's reward system, which enhances bonding. Our biology contributes to an intrinsic motivation to affiliate with others and be socially engaged. Becoming **I am Interconnected** has a biological foundation.

This strong mind-body need is belongingness, our human emotional need to be an accepted member of a group. Our need to belong encourages us to seek out stable, long-lasting relationships with other groups of people. This natural desire to belong and be an important part of something greater than ourselves motivates us to participate in social activities such as clubs, sports teams, religious groups, and community organizations. Recent discoveries in science point to supportive relationships as the most robust predictor of positive attributes such as longevity, medical and mental health, happiness and even wisdom across our lifespan.

Contributing in groups can be mutually beneficial for every member of the group as well as those we serve. We increase our satisfaction and excel when have a role and function that invites us to utilize our gifts, talents, and passions. Imagine a fish measuring its success by its capacity to climb a tree. The fish carries the same inner essence as all living being, and has distinct ways of being in the world. Through awareness, research, and contemplation, we realize more deeply our innate tendencies and preferences. When we live as our whole and Holy self, we radiate our passion and catalyze transformation. As the Bhagavad Gita (Chapter 18, verse 47) reminds us:

Better is one's own duty destitute of merits, than the duty of another well performed. Doing the duty ordained according to nature one incurs no sin.[21]

Contributing at work, whether volunteer or paid, matters to us and the organization. We can feel unsatisfied if this need to belong and contribute is not met. Limiting or false beliefs of scarcity inside ourselves or an organizational culture stuck in **I am Individual** can sabotage fulfillment at work. When we bring our awareness to our ideas of lack, we have the choice to release them and shift into abundance and live in **I am Interconnected** and **I am Infinite.** Are any of these limiting beliefs present in your work?

- It's not safe
- You can't make a difference
- There is not enough
- It needs to be hard and a struggle to be worth something
- You don't deserve ease and flow
- People are disposable
- You are waiting for someone else to improve your workplace
- You need to play small to be acceptable
- Your value is determined by other people's perceptions
- You can't change

---

21   Ben-Ami Scharfstein, *Mystical Experience* (Indianapolis: Bobbs-Merrill, 1973).

- You are not worthy

- You are not ready to be seen

We can embody wholeness and Holiness even if the culture of our organization and some of the individuals who participate in it operate from **I am Individual.** We can set the tone and culture for our teams. We can be a leader, who is anyone committed to service and enhancing their organization. Whether we have formal leadership titles or not, we are called to engage fully in our workgroups in higher consciousness.

We are invited to create a sacred space where each person is encouraged to produce for the highest good. Our tone or vibe of integrity, vulnerability, authenticity, openness, and flexibility are mirrored in our teams. When we operate primarily from being whole and Holy we are more resilient. We recognize quickly when we are out of alignment and can return to balance with ease and flow.

When we are clear and calm, we can feel the subtle energies. As leaders, this gives us the ability to know and understand shifts and changes in ourselves and in our teams as they occur in the present moment. We can follow and create openings of resonance, aliveness, and coherence. We gain clarity in visioning what next steps best serve the mission. We are able to pay attention and notice solutions and details of how to best proceed. This encourages everyone in our group to access their genius, innovation and creativity. It is a gift for us as leaders to give our team members a safe place to be their best selves. Together we co-create and attract our future with an energy that is expansive, trusting, and brilliant.

When you as a leader embody whole and Holy leadership:

- You recognize synchronicity, patterns, and subtle energy
- You recognize the patterns, ease and flow in systems
- You empower others to take their own initiative
- You recognize people's undeveloped skills, strengths talents and encourage this inner capacity
- You create a safe space which supports healing and wholeness
- Your creativity and inspiration flows and encourage others
- You shift easily between an expansive perspective and key details
- You are an authentic communicator, both in speaking and listening
- You set clear intentions, goals, and outcomes
- You manifest and create
- You are kind
- You are a catalyst of transformation and change
- You are receptive, accepting what comes to you that nurtures and supports you
- Your presence is felt by others
- You are personally and mutually accountable
- You see clearly what is actually occurring
- You recognize opportunities for growth and improvement and lead towards those openings

- You have clear thought and speech
- You are flexible inside a solid structure
- You are comfortable with change
- You are productive and have abundant energy
- You are efficient and effective

Leadership from a lived whole and Holy worldview has direct impact on all parts of the organization and team. As I mentioned in chapter two, I had managed a division for a national healthcare company. My leadership improved as I shifted into knowing myself as a larger part of the sea of consciousness. I had less need to control, protect, and micromanage my team. I was more open to intuitive creative solutions. I could feel the micro-changes that would best serve us as we moved towards our intended outcomes.

We developed the strengths of our staff. We revised our processes to enhance efficiency and effectiveness. Each person on our team was more engaged in our business. Our patient care improved. Our division became more successful in both human and financial performance. Our sales grew, our variable expenses decreased, our profit margin increased, our turnover rate declined, and we had less sick days. We improved our top and bottom line. As business transforms, we are more often measuring and valuing a triple bottom line which includes social, environmental (or ecological) and financial aspects of our organizations.

As I expanded my awareness, my leaders and their staff became more accountable, empowered, collaborative, and productive. We all improved our ability to work under stress, run meetings, manage time, and delegate. We enhanced their capacity to make decisions and identify the root causes of issues and implement timely and effective solutions. I found two key components were fundamental to all of the improvements: more trust and better communication.

Research on the mind-body connection demonstrates how important building trust is when contributing in the world. Human beings have hardwired systems exquisitely designed to let us know where we stand with others. Based on a quick read of a situation, our brains know whether we should operate in a protective mode or be open to sharing, discovery, and influence. As we learned in chapter ten, sensory information is received and gets sorted through a region of the limbic system called the thalamus. The information gets relayed along two pathways simultaneously. One is a short pathway, that involves no thinking, to the amygdala, a region of the limbic system. The second is a longer pathway to the cortex.

If we determine we are in a threatening situation and it is perceived we are not safe, the brain automatically activates the fight, flight or freeze response. We only have access to our brainstem, which is instinctual and focused on survival. When our conversations are subject to this lockdown, we get more "stuck" in our point of view. Protecting ourselves is hardwired in our brains. Fear and conflict not only change the chemistry of the brains, they also change how we feel, how we behave, and how others perceive us. In a nanosecond we can move from being seen as a trusted friend and advisor to being seen as a frightening threat, a person distrusted. We diminish our capacity to effectively lead and contribute in the world.

Invitation to Practice

- Find a quiet place to relax and close your eyes. Take a few deep breaths. Feel your feet on the ground and your body supported, alert, and calm.

- Call to mind a group you belong to that is important to you. Feel the gratitude you have for this group's presence in your life. Allow that sensation of appreciation and connection to permeate your heart, mind, and body.

- When you participate in this group, how do you contribute from your Divine Essence?

- Are there ways you can enhance your communication and build more trust?

- How can you cultivate your group's creativity, connection, and joy?

- Send a blessing of thankfulness to each member of the group, including yourself.

On the other side of the brain spectrum is the cortex. This is the newest brain, and it enables us to build societies, have good judgment, be strategic, handle difficult conversations, and build and sustain trust. Here we process incoming information with full access to our capacity for speech, higher order thinking, sensory perception, witness perspective and cognizant thought. When input is not deemed dangerous, we complete the path to the cortex and we are capable of responding instead of reacting. We are able to grow and expand instead of closing down. When we feel safe, we cultivate satisfaction and connection. When we are contributing in the world it is essential to cultivate trust.

We can cultivate trust, communicate authentically, empathize, and remain calm even if those around us are stressed and reactive. I had an opportunity to practice these skills working in a community pharmacy. A man walked up to the pharmacy counter to pick up his mother's insulin. The prescription was not filled, and he began to yell at my technician to find out why it was not ready. As he escalated, she glanced my way, inviting me to assist.

I walked over to relieve her, and he recapped his demand to get the insulin immediately. I took a deep breath, in through my nose and out through my mouth, which activated the relaxation response in my mind-body. I utilized all five of my senses to bring my awareness more fully into the moment. What was he saying behind the words? I opened my ears and eyes fully. Clearly he was frustrated beyond the presenting circumstances. He felt confused and in pain. What did I feel in my body? I opened my heart to connect with his. I felt centered, feeling the bottoms of my feet planted firmly on the ground.

After every few sentences, I mirrored his words to demonstrate understanding. My technician's search of our database showed that his mother's prescription had been filled and picked up a few days earlier at another pharmacy nearby. He loudly told me that was impossible, and I would be responsible for his mother's uncontrolled diabetes and potential death if I did not give him the medicine immediately. I offered to give it to him. It would be $100 as the insurance would not pay for a refill so soon after the medication was picked up. He escalated. I mirrored.

I had one of my technicians call the other pharmacy to confirm it had indeed been picked up. Yes, they had an electronic image of the signature verifying it had been picked up. He was livid. They were lying. I had them fax me the signature. I assured him we would find a solution that would not leave his mother without her life sustaining medications. While waiting and conversing, he began to lower his voice a bit, explaining he was on his way to pick up his mother for a doctor's appointment and was on a very tight timeline.

The fax arrived, and I presented it to him. He began to tear up. The signature was his father's. He explained his dad was suffering from Alzheimer's disease and must have picked up the insulin a few days prior at the other pharmacy near their home and did not remember. The man went on to share that his mother has been the full time caregiver for his father, and they were still living together in their home. With her diabetes and other health problems worsening, she had been in and out of the hospital and his caring for his aging parents had become unmanageable. He looked me in the eyes and offered a thank you and an apology. He would find the insulin in his parent's home before heading to the doctor's appointment. I looked into eyes, connecting to his **Center Within**. I assured him his apology was accepted and wished him and his family well.

These same skills translate into any group of which we are a part. Family is another primary place we satisfy our need for belonging and contributing. Often families, like organizations, have dysfunctional patterns that roll from one generation to the next. When we transform our perspective to **I am Interconnected** and **I am Infinite**, we bring the gift of higher awareness, choice and freedom to our families. We bring peace to those who came before us and spare the generations that follow. In my own family, my generation of siblings has chosen to be more open, loving, and supportive than the family we were raised in.

Bo Lozoff, an American writer and interfaith humanitarian, reminds us that contributing to our daily events and encounters from our **Center Within** matters:

> There is no spiritual practice more profound than being kind to one's family and neighbors, the cashier at the grocery store, an unexpected visitor, a stray cat or dog, or any other of the usually irrelevant and invisible beings who may cross our paths in the course of a normal day. Certainly there are spiritual mysteries to explore, but as we mature it becomes clear that those special experiences are only meaningful when they arise from and return to ordinary kindness.[22]

In my family, our ability to be of service and contribute to our mutual benefit was put to the test when my father died. In both of my parent's families, there was conflict, distrust, and division that occurred between siblings when their second parent died. We intended that pattern of destruction to end with us.

---

22   Bo Lozoff, *It's a Meaningful Life: It Just Takes Practice* (New York: Penguin Compass, 2001).

Dad called on a Sunday afternoon to say he was not feeling well. My sister who lived the closest stopped in to check on him. His COPD (chronic obstructive pulmonary disease) had taken a turn for the worse and he was frustrated and depressed. My siblings and I took turns staying with dad continuously for the next three days. My brother and brother-in-law took the Tuesday evening shift. My father died in his bed with my brother holding his hand.

Our ability to be in the present moment, be with my father, be with each other, and be with what was actually occurring was astounding. There was no drama, no minimizing his rapidly declining condition, no blame, no judgment, no regrets. We allowed space for each other to grieve in our own ways. Could we maintain this level of kindness and connection, allowing each of us to have our own opinions and process while unexpectedly settling his affairs?

All the years of my practice in authentic communication, organizational development, spiritual and transforming practices and coaching converged within me as I navigated my way through the process. We had the house to sell and contents to sort, divide, and donate. The house needed some repairs and updates, but which ones and how many? We are four successful independent self-sufficient adults (at least we think so!) who all make decisions differently and have diverse priorities.

As the process unfolded, we continued to remain open and honest. When an issue came up where we felt stuck, we stopped our forging ahead and connected. We got clear about the issue, listened, reflected, and resolved the small differences of opinion before continuing. We often felt vulnerable and chose to remain transparent. We found it most effective if the person needing more time or information took the lead, did the research, and presented their preferences. From finding the best value for redoing the hardwood floors, to meticulously sorting out the contents of the garage, to which areas of the house we would replace the paint and carpet, to setting the price to sell and adjusting it in a volatile home value market, we found consensus with everyone's voice each step of the way. We emerged from the process feeling heard and supported. Each of us felt more trust and connection.

Resolving conflict is an art and a science. When we participate on teams, whether at work, volunteer organizations, or in our family or community, our ability to contribute is directly influenced by our capacity to effectively settle disagreements. It is important to maintain a spirit of nurturance, affirmation and cooperation. In effective conflict resolution, we decide what we are willing to do or give to make the situation better. We do not force, coerce or pressure the other person to do it our way. We make conflict resolution into an esteem-building and trust-enhancing process rather than a negative and destructive one.

We are invited to bring our whole, Holy, and awake self to every moment. There will be moments we find that our inner state of overarousal or irritation does not readily support mindful contributing. There may be times we drop back into doubt, worry, reactivity, or judgement. Our outer world and circumstances can bring chaos and drama. When we slide back into lower consciousness, we practice bringing our attention back into the present moment.

We do not accept bad behavior, violence or others imposing immature ideals on each other. We do not allow destruction by greed or intolerance. We are moved to heal the wounds of separation in our own minds and hearts, in our families and communities, and in the world. We practice mindfulness and heartfulness.

When we are at peace in moments of inner or outer disruption, we invite others to attune their mirror neurons to our calm energy. Each of us emits a vibration in every moment, affecting all seen and unseen life in the sea of consciousness. When we contribute living as **I am Infinite**, life around us matches our frequency like a tuning fork. Our very presence impacts change. We are invited to embody and live the change that we desire in the world. Our very presence manifesting as me, we, and Thee expressing in the world, catalyzes transformation.

Reflection

Is there a person at your work who sets the culture or tone? Is he or she empowering or disempowering? What characteristics and behaviors does he or she demonstrate that influence the rest of the team?

In your family, are you honest and direct with one another? Do you create sacred space for each person to be heard and valued? Do you resolve conflict as it arises?

How do you build trust and connection in your groups?

What are your inherent strengths and passions that align with and support your service in the world?

How do you remain in your **Center Within** when there is chaos in a group you belong to?

CHAPTER FOURTEEN

IMAGINING OUR FUTURE

You are invited to embody higher consciousness and be in the world as an everyday mystic as we usher in this new era of humanity and co-create who we are becoming.

We are living during a time of tremendous growth and transformation. We understand that expanding our awareness, focusing our attention, and clarifying our intention cultivates openings to higher consciousness. This opportunity is available for all human beings. We each have the ability to realize our full potential. What would our world look like if every individual, every relationship, and every family, institution, community and organization shifted into higher consciousness? Let's envision the possibilities.

For eons, being aware of and avoiding danger has been a critical survival skill for human beings. Our brains were hardwired to emphasize the negative rather than the positive. We made choices based on our need to avoid harmful experiences. We can understand our human history while making different choices for ourselves. A shift could look like us knowing and expressing our genius. We could spend our resources like time, money, and intention developing and expressing our gifts, wisdom and compassion in the world. With our needs met, we could love our whole and Holy self, and feel satisfied. We could create and serve from our passions, interests and strengths because it biologically positions us beyond surviving to thriving.

Scientists are discovering new genes arising out of so-called junk DNA, or non-coding DNA. They are the mysterious stretches of DNA between known genes. Scientists are seeing new genetic function somehow spring into existence.[23] I imagine these genes becoming active in response to the higher vibration radiating into the field as we shift into higher consciousness. I imagine these genes are expressing now to support innate capacities which have been dormant at our previous levels of development. As more people open themselves to **I am Infinite** awareness and live in higher consciousness, we contribute to raising the vibration of the collective field of consciousness. This morphic resonance is shared with all beings. Every individual shift creates a higher frequency for the whole. This allows easier access to higher levels of consciousness for all humans.

Remember the spiral path humanity is traveling on? We are at the end of a long gradual ascent, whipping around the outer edge of a sharp curve moving us towards another long gradual ascent at a higher level. There is tremendous speed

---

23. Emily Singer, "A Surprise Source of Life's Code," *Quanta Magazine,* August 31, 2015, www.scientificamerican.com/article/a-surprise-source-of-life-s-code/?WT.mc_id=SA_WR_20150902.

around the curve of a spiral. When nature reaches a limitation, it innovates and transforms, evolving towards higher consciousness and more freedom. This quantum leap in development creates intense possibilities, opportunities, and conditions for new perspectives and capacities to emerge. I imagine we can perceive new areas in the field of consciousness. Our perceptivity to subtle ways of knowing increases. Multiple types of intelligence are expanding including telepathy, clairvoyance, and intuition. We flourish as our interconnectedness is known in our bodies at a cellular level.

One way to imagine this is to picture a piano. We have known the piano to have a certain number of keys, representing the field of consciousness. With this passage in human history, the piano keyboard we will be playing on is larger and more expanded than before. It may have more octaves of high and low notes, or even various levels of keys. We will be able to create music never before possible with access to the keys previously unavailable as they were beyond our perception.

I visualize the spectrum of sound waves we know exist all around us. We are like receivers and are able to tune into the various frequencies. Humans have been able to perceive certain tones on the continuum of sound while others are outside of the range of what we can hear. If our capacities as receivers improve, we will be able to pick up a larger range of sound with more ease. Our perceptive mechanisms themselves are progressing. The field of consciousness is not changing, nor is the spectrum of sound waves. It is our ability to hear, to send and receive signals that is changing. Imagine our current hardware is being upgraded and new software is being downloaded. Our ways of knowing are being enhanced.

Invitation to Practice

- Take a deep breath in through your nose and out through your mouth. Feel your belly soften and expand. Repeat three times.

- Invite a sense of gratitude for creating the time to read today. What a gift you have given yourself. Feel it in your heart.

- Allow that sense of appreciation to spread to your entire body.

- Feel your connection to the field of consciousness. Imagine supportive energy flowing in your body and enhancing every cell. Linger in this openness as each cell is upgraded.

- Take a few minutes to relax further into this sensation of gratitude and high vibration.

- When you are ready, return your attention to your breath. Wiggle your fingers and toes.

The shift toward higher consciousness changes what we value in relationships. As we are no longer dependent on others to fill our holes, we can nurture relationships that mutually support our potential being realized. We call each other forward into our genius, our whole and Holy selves. We choose partners to encourage the development of each other's strengths and passions. We cultivate relationships with people who inspire us and enhance our sense of belonging. We are increasingly sensitive to the energy of others while maintaining our own centeredness. We are more compassionate, able to be with one another in joy and sorrow, without any need to fix or judge.

When the outdated belief that differences in people are a threat no longer exists, individuals and organizations that previously justified their self-centered focus of oppression are transformed. I imagine in our new era that diversity will be valued as a necessity and we will see ourselves as global citizens. Solidarity prevails. I wonder what a flag that represents one humanity would look like.

I imagine a worldwide system with members from every country who identify areas of need. Resources are directed with ease towards relieving suffering and restoring the distressed areas to balance and wholeness. Groups emerge from this integrated worldwide system that work together on new inventions and discoveries. Technology would be used to support the greater good, arising from a higher level of understanding, wisdom, and compassion. There would be teams that coalesce to form innovation hubs and pool resources to create new life-sustaining inventions and structures to assure the basic needs of all beings are met. Creation would flourish under such support. Solutions previously outside of our comprehension would emerge from the larger field of consciousness we now perceive.

In our new era, we will find like-minded and like-hearted people to collaborate with on projects that make our heart sing.

Our inherent drive to contribute through expressing our gifts, passions, and strengths guide us to serve. Complacency and unnecessary dependency would cease to exist.

At a higher level of consciousness, we demand transparency and are intolerant of obscuring or distorting the truth. If we relapse into greed, it quickly becomes exposed and we readjust to the new era norm of authenticity and openness. We remember that we are all interconnected, and we value that which is mutually beneficial. We remember we are and have enough.

The value of products and services would be measured by how well they support living cells. This includes cells in our bodies, the environment, and in all beings living on the planet. Our policies globally from industries to institutions are aligned with these standards. Innovation in every area holds cell health as the highest measure of success and development. Information on all products' enhancement of cell health would be readily available.

Companies would actively identify employee's talents and hire people into positions that match their strengths. Employees are more engaged, productive, and creative because they work in jobs that utilize their gifts. The goal of a strong organization is to maximize each person's potential. It is a place to innovate and express each person's inner nature. I imagine leaders who successfully cultivate higher levels of consciousness in themselves, their teams and the organizations. This capacity would be rewarded financially and highly developed leaders are provided more opportunities to expand their influence. Every worker and the organization thrive.

I imagine education systems that support each student's expression of his or her innate genius. Education is available to all children. Every student would be competent in the full array of intelligences including social, emotional, physical, spiritual, financial, integral, interpersonal, logical, environmental, musical, artistic, linguistic, and existential intelligence before they leave high school. Every student would be aware of their strengths and gifts and have tools to continue developing them. Being a lifelong learner would be valued and encouraged.

Cosmology, our understanding of the large scale view of the universe as a whole, is also changing as we embrace higher consciousness. There is new wisdom revealing itself as we embody expanded levels of awareness and compassion. As this evolutionary surge completes itself over time, I believe we will be radically different than who we know ourselves to be today. This will be a quantum leap in access to a higher level of consciousness for humanity as a whole. All aspects of life, from the arts to government, from economics to health, from culture to families, will reflect this shift.

At this moment, we are writing the next book in our history on planet earth. Our mythology, the stories of humanity that contain our ideals, values, traditions, and beliefs are built on our history. Our previous stories are being honored as we write our new stories from an expanding worldview. I invite you to embody higher consciousness, and be in the world as an everyday mystic as we usher in this new era of humanity and co-create who we are becoming.

Reflection

In your professional or volunteer life, what changes can you imagine that would reflect serving from **I am Infinite?**

How would your body, mind, and emotions shift if you fully embodied higher consciousness?

What relationships in your life cultivate higher consciousness?

What are the three most impactful ideas in this book? How have they influenced your life? How will you continue to deepen and embody the principles in yourself, your relationships and your work?

What would an ideal planet look like when we leave it to those who will inherit the earth?

RESOURCES FOR STAGES OF CONSCIOUSNESS

Don Edward Beck and Christopher Cowan, *Spiral Dynamics: Mastering Values, Leadership, and Change* (Malden: Blackwell Publishing, 1996).

Deepak Chopra, *How to Know God: The Soul's Journey into the Mystery of the Mysteries* (New York: Harmony Books, 2000).

John Davis, *The Diamond Approach: An Introduction to the Teachings of A.H. Almaas* (Boston: Shambhala Publications, Inc., 1999).

Wayne Dyer, *You'll See it When You Believe It: The Way to Your Personal Transformation* (New York: HarperCollins Publishers, 1989).

Jean Hardy, *Psychology with a Soul: Psychosynthesis in Evolutionary Content* (New York: Penguin Books, 1987).

David Hawkins, *Power vs. Force: The Hidden Determinants of Human Behavior* (Carlsbad: Hay House, 2002).

Abraham Maslow, *Motivation and Personality* (New York: Harper & Row, 1970).

Ken Wilbur, *The Integral Vision: An Introduction to the Revolutionary Integral Approach to Life, God, the Universe and Everything* (Boston: Shambhala Publications, 2007).

MORE RESOURCES

Websites

Center for Consciousness Studies (http://consciousness.arizona.edu)

Center for Healthy Minds (http://centerhealthyminds.org/)

The Center for Mind-Body Medicine (http://www.cmbm.org/)

Center for Spirituality & Healing, U of MN (http://www.csh.umn.edu/)

Greater Good: The Science of a Meaningful Life (http://greatergood. berkeley.edu)

HeartMath™ (http://www.heartmath.org/)

The Institute of Noetic Sciences (http://noetic.org/)

The Integral Institute (http://www.integralinstitute.org/)

The Optimist Magazine (http://www.theoptimist.com/magazine/)

Science and NonDuality (https://www.scienceandnonduality.com)

Books (in addition to the references cited throughout the book)

Herbert Benson, *The Relaxation Response* (New York: Morrow, 1975).

Gregg Braden, *The Divine Matrix: Bridging Time, Space, Miracles and Belief* (Carlsbad: Hay House, 2007).

Larry Dossey, *One Mind: How our Individual Mind is Part of a Greater Consciousness and Why it Matters* (Carlsbad: Hay House, 2013).

Henry Emmons, M.D., *Staying Sharp: 9 Keys for a Youthful Brain Through Modern Science and Ageless Wisdom* (New York: Touchstone, 2015).

Astrid Fitzgerald, *Being Consciousness Bliss: A Seeker's Guide* (Great Barrington: Lindisfarne Books, 2001).

Daniel Goleman, *Emotional Intelligence: Why it Can Matter More Than IQ* (New York: Bantam, 2005).

Jon Kabat-Zinn, *Full Catastrophe Living: Using the Wisdom of Your Body and Mind to Face Stress, Pain and Illness* (New York: Dell, 1991).

Bruce Lipton, PhD., *The Biology of Belief: Unleashing the Power of Consciousness, Matter and Miracles* (Carlsbad: Hay House, 2008).

Barbara Marx Hubbard, *Conscious Evolution: Awakening the Power of our Social Potential* (Novato: New World Library, 1998).

David Perlmutter M.D. & Alberto Villoldo, *Power up Your Brain: The Neuroscience of Enlightenment* (New York: Hay House, 2011).

Daniel J. Siegel, M.D., *Mindsight: The New Science of Personal Transformation* (New York: Bantam, 2010).

Amit Sood, M.D., MSc., *The Mayo Clinic Guide to Stress-Free Living* (Cambridge: Da Capo Lifelong Books, 2013).

INDEX